TABLE OF C

Top 20 Test Taking Tips

1. Carefully follow all the test registration procedures
2. Know the test directions, duration, topics, question types, how many questions
3. Setup a flexible study schedule at least 3-4 weeks before test day
4. Study during the time of day you are most alert, relaxed, and stress free
5. Maximize your learning style; visual learner use visual study aids, auditory learner use auditory study aids
6. Focus on your weakest knowledge base
7. Find a study partner to review with and help clarify questions
8. Practice, practice, practice
9. Get a good night's sleep; don't try to cram the night before the test
10. Eat a well balanced meal
11. Know the exact physical location of the testing site; drive the route to the site prior to test day
12. Bring a set of ear plugs; the testing center could be noisy
13. Wear comfortable, loose fitting, layered clothing to the testing center; prepare for it to be either cold or hot during the test
14. Bring at least 2 current forms of ID to the testing center
15. Arrive to the test early; be prepared to wait and be patient
16. Eliminate the obviously wrong answer choices, then guess the first remaining choice
17. Pace yourself; don't rush, but keep working and move on if you get stuck
18. Maintain a positive attitude even if the test is going poorly
19. Keep your first answer unless you are positive it is wrong
20. Check your work, don't make a careless mistake

Gather Nutrition Data

Common dietary abbreviations

Some commonly encountered abbreviations that may appear in the dietary notes of a medical chart include the following:
- ac - Before meal(s)
- bid - Twice per day
- BMI - Body Mass Index
- c - With
- CHO - Carbohydrate
- gr - Grain
- hs - At bedtime
- liq - Liquid
- MDR - Minimum daily requirement
- Na - Sodium
- NPO - Nothing by mouth
- p - After
- pc - After meal(s)
- po - By mouth
- PRO - protein
- qid - Four times per day
- TBW - Total body weight
- TF - Tube feedings
- tid - Three times per day
- wt - Weight

Nutritional assessment form

The nutritional assessment form is called the Minimum Data Set (MDS). MDS is a patient overview/history that is included in the medical chart. The MDS assesses every aspect (physical, social, psychological, emotional, et cetera) of a patient's status. Included in the MDS is a brief overview (Section AC) followed by a lengthy listing of questions regarding a patient's history. In addition to the questions regarding a patient's eating patterns in Section AC, an in-depth assessment of oral and nutritional health appears in Section K. That assessment includes questions regarding intake, weight gain or loss, ability to taste, problems chewing or swallowing, and the use of feeding devices such as tube and intravenous feeding supplements.

Medical chart

Medical charts must be maintained with the highest regard to precision and accuracy. Because many medical personnel may be accessing the chart on a daily basis, it is important that documents be placed in the correct section of the medical record and that notes are clearly and legibly written. Dietary information is most often found in the dietary section and/or progress notes section of a medical chart. Additionally, the nutritional assessment form, called the minimum data set, is also an important document to reference. Be careful to document all notes, progress reports, and recommendations accurately and legibly, always in blue or black (preferred) ink. When a change is necessary, using an ink pen, draw a single line through the text. Do not scribble or completely block out the previously written notes. Some facilities also require that all revisions are initialed.

Diet history

A diet history is essential to determining the current nutritional habits of a client and developing an ongoing nutritional plan for the individual(s). A diet history should include information about the client's daily intake, disabilities and/or conditions that may impede the client's ability to consume various types of food, ethnic and cultural influences (flavoring, food staples, prohibited foods), and religious restrictions (meals must be kosher, does not eat meat, seasonal food restrictions, etc). Additionally, it is important to inquire about allergies, drug therapies (some foods may interfere with drug absorption and/or pharmaceuticals may alter tastes), sense of taste and smell, and appetite. When taking a diet history, it may be helpful to employ recording methods such as utilizing a 3-day food record, administering a food frequency questionnaire, and interviewing the client (as well as his/her caretaker, if applicable). When interviewing a client regarding his/her diet history, it is important to do so in a manner that is neither leading nor intimidating to the client. If the client is not a native English speaker, arrange for a translator to assist with the interview. Likewise, if the client is unable to communicate and/or is suffering from memory loss/dementia, it is advisable to have a family member or other caretaker present at the interview. When asking questions, be aware of phrasing so as to avoid leading a client to answer in a manner that would appease the interviewer. For example, instead of asking, "You don't eat dessert at every meal, do you?" You may ask, "Approximately how many servings of sweets (to include cookies, cakes, puddings, pies, etc) do you eat daily?" Finally, watch for nonverbal cues from the client. Consistent head-nodding may indicate that the individual does not fully understand the question or language used. Lack of eye contact and focus may be a sign that the client is not alert or that he/she may be confused.

Measurements and tests

Anthropometric measurements
Anthropometric measurements are comparative body measurements that may be used to help determine whether a client is growing at a healthy rate, weight loss or gain has occurred, and/or to have a baseline value off of which to implement dietary, pharmaceutical, and/or physical activity changes. These measurements are generally included in the nutritional assessment. Anthropometric measurements are measurements of one's physical traits, and they include height, weight, waist-to-hip ratio, head circumference (in infants), body density, body mass index and other similar measurements that assess weight, growth, and development. When assessing anthropometric measurements, one must take the utmost care and have precision as small measurement errors can cause great assessment variations.

Biochemical tests

Urinalyses and blood draws provide data necessary for biochemical tests. Most often, these tests are used to detect visceral protein levels, which may be derived from serum albumin, transferrin, and prealbumin. Tests may be useful in measuring hemoglobin and glucose levels. Biochemical tests may also be used to determine levels of various vitamins and minerals, such as iron, present in the body. Biochemical tests are often considered part of a nutritional assessment. However, many factors, including stress, surgery, hydration, and functioning of internal organs (especially kidneys and liver) may alter test values. Thus, biochemical tests must be evaluated in light of other nutritional assessments such as anthropometric measurements, diet journals, clinical visits, as well as social and medical histories.

Nutritional assessment

A nutritional assessment is performed to determine the nutritional needs and habits of a client. The assessment may be essential to finding and understanding dietary deficiencies or excesses as well as to formulation of a nutritional plan for a client. Nutritional assessments most often incorporate a variety of data, which assess physical and biochemical traits, dietary habits, and psychosocial well-being. Physical traits are evaluated through the use of anthropometric measurements, including height, weight, and body mass index, among others. Biochemical tests are used to assess protein, vitamin, and mineral deficiencies. Psychosocial assessments help the practitioner determine whether depression, lack of social interaction, or other factors may influence a client's dietary habits. When performing and evaluating a nutritional assessment, it is imperative that all parts of the assessment are considered. Daily dietary changes, life stresses, hydration levels, and medical therapies may all skew individual tests results and clinical presentation.

Clinical data help round out the nutritional assessment picture. Such data may include medical and treatment histories as well as any current treatment information. Life stresses, medical treatments, including surgeries, therapies, and pharmaceutical interventions, over-the-counter medicine use, and daily routine may all affect one's nutritional status. Absorption of key nutrients is frequently impeded or altered by drug therapies and life stresses. As with all parts of the nutritional assessment, the clinical data must be evaluated by a professional and in accordance to information gleaned from other data, such as anthropometric measurements, biochemical tests, diet journal, and patient history.

Calculating weight change

Suppose a client typically weighs 175 lbs, however, his current body weight is 145 lbs. To calculate percent weight change, you must identify the original weight, W_1 (175 lbs) and the current weight, W_2 (145 lbs). Subtract the current weight from the original weight, W_1-W_2. Divide that product by the original weight, so that $(W_1-W_2)/W_1$. Now, multiply the product by 100. So that, $[(W_1-W_2)/W_1]$ x 100 equals percent weight change. In the case of this example:
- [(175 lbs-145 lbs)/175 lbs x 100 = percent weight change
- [(30 lbs)/175 lbs] x 100 = percent weight change
- [0.171] x 100 = percent weight change
- 17.1 = percent weight change

Harris-Benedict Equation

The Harris-Benedict Equation is often used to determine one's energy requirements, and thus, a goal caloric intake. The equation utilizes one's basal metabolic rate (BMR) in combination with activity levels to determine energy requirement values. To determine a client's daily caloric requirement, use one of the following equations:
- Sedentary: Caloric requirement = 1.2 x BMR
- Mildly active (mild exercise 1-3 times weekly): Caloric requirement = 1.375 x BMR
- Moderately active (moderate exercise, 3-5 times weekly): Caloric requirement = 1.55 x BMR
- Very active (hard exercise, 6-7 times weekly): Caloric requirement = 1.725 x BMR
- Excessively active (very hard exercise, 2-a-day training): Caloric requirement = 1.9 x BMR

BMR

BMR is the acronym for basal metabolic rate. This value quantifies one's metabolic rate and is used in the Harris-Benedict Equation to determine a client's energy requirements. To calculate the basal metabolic rate (BMR), use the following equations:
- WOMEN: BRM = 655 + (9.6 x weight in kilograms) + (1.8 x height in centimeters) – (4.7 x age in years)
- MEN: BRM = 66 + (13.7 x weight in kilograms) + (5 x height in centimeters) – (6.8 x age in years)

Converting units of measurement

Pounds: To convert pounds to kilograms the conversion is 1 pound = 0.45 kilograms. To determine how many kilograms a 135 lbs woman weighs, use the following equation:
- Pounds x 0.454 = Kilograms
- 135 lbs x 0.454 kg/lb = 61.29 kg

Ounces to grams: To convert ounces to grams the conversion is 1 ounce = 28.35 grams. To determine how many grams are in 3.5 ounces, use the following equation:
- Ounces x 28.35 = Grams
- 3.5 oz x 28.35 g/oz = 99.23 g

Grams: There are 1000 grams in a kilogram. To convert grams to kilograms, divide by 1000 or move the decimal three places to the left. So that 99.23 grams equals .09923 kilograms. Conversely, to convert kilograms to grams, multiply by 1000 or move the decimal three places to the right, so that 99.23 kilograms equals 99230 grams.

Feet: To convert feet to meters the conversion is 1 foot = 0.3048 meters. To determine how many meters a 5'6" woman is, use the following equation:
- Feet x 0.3048 = Meters
- 5.5 ft x 0.3048 m/ft =1.68 m

Inches: To convert inches to centimeters the conversion is 1 inch = 2.54 centimeters. To determine how many centimeters a 5'6" woman is, use the following equation:
- Inches x 2.54 = Centimeters (Remember, there are 12 inches in every foot)
- 66 in x 2.54 cm/in = 167.64 cm

Centimeters: There are 100 centimeters in every meter. To convert centimeters to meters, divide by 100 or move the decimal two places to the left. So that 167.64 cm equals 1.6764 m. Conversely, to convert meters to centimeters, multiply by 100 or move the decimal two places to the right, so that 1.67 m equals 167 centimeters.

Ounces to milliliters: One ounce is equivalent to 29.57 milliliters. Use the following equation to convert six ounces to milliliters:
- 6 oz x 29.57 mL/oz = 177.42 mL

Cups to liters: Likewise, one cup is equal to 0.237 liters. Use the following equation to convert one and a third cups to liters:
- 1.33 c x 0.237 L/c = .315 L

There are 1000 milliliters in a liter. Therefore, to convert milliliters to liters, divide by 1000 or move the decimal three spaces to the left so that 177.42 mL equals 0.177 L. Conversely, to convert liters to milliliters, multiply by 1000 or move the decimal three places to the right, so that .315 L equals 315 mL.
**Note: One milliliter is equivalent to one cubic centimeter.

Calculating body mass index (BMI)

To calculate body mass index of a woman who weighs 135 lbs and stands 5'6" tall, first convert pounds to kilograms and inches to meters. So, 135 lbs x 0.454 lb/kg = 61.29 kg and (66 in x 2.54 cm/in)/100 = 1.68 m.

Now, use the following equation to calculate BMI:
- BMI = (Weight in kilograms) / (Height in meters)(Height in meters)
- •BMI = (Weight in kilograms) / (Height in meters)^2
- BMI = (61.29 kg) /(1.68 m) ^{2}
- BMI = (61.29 kg) / (2.82 m^2)
- BMI = 21.72 kg/m^2

** Note, the non-metric BMI formula is as follows:
- BMI = [(Weight in pounds) / (Height in inches) ^{2}] x 703

Ideal body weight

For medium framed males, the ideal body weight (IBW) at five feet (60 inches) is 106 lbs. For every inch greater than 60 inches, add six pounds. So, to calculate the ideal body weight for a 6'3" medium framed male, use the following equation:
- Convert feet to inches: 6 ft (12 in/ft) + 3 in = 75 in

Now calculate IBW:
- (75 in - 60 in)(6lbs/in) + 106 lbs = 196 lbs

Likewise, for medium framed females, the ideal body weight at five feet (60 inches) is 100 lbs. For every inch greater than 60 inches, add five pounds. Use the same set-up as above, substituting the new values to calculate a 5'7" woman's IBW:

- Convert feet to inches: 5 ft (12 in/ft) + 7 in = 67 in

Now calculate IBW:

- (67 in – 60 in)(5 lbs/in) +100 lbs = 135 lbs

Percentage of ideal body weight

A 5'9" male patient weighs 137 lbs. To calculate the percentage of ideal body weight (IBW), first determine a client's ideal body weight:

- IBW for a male = 106 lbs + (height in inches – 60 in)(6 lbs)
- IBW for this patient = 106 lbs + (69 in -60 in)(6 lbs)
- IBW = 106 lbs + 54 lbs = 160 lbs.

Now calculate percentage of ideal body weight by dividing the current weight by the ideal weight and multiply by 100, so that:

- % IBW = (137 lbs / 160 lbs) x 100
- % IBW = 85.63%

Vitamins and nutrients

<u>MyPlate</u>
The USDA's Food Pyramid was heavily criticized for being vague and confusing, and in 2011 it was replaced with MyPlate. MyPlate is much easier to understand, as it consists of a picture of a dinner plate divided into four sections, visually illustrating how our daily diet should be distributed among the various food groups. Vegetables and grains each take up 30% of the plate, while fruits and proteins each constitute 20% of the plate. There is also a representation of a cup, marked Dairy, alongside the plate. The idea behind MyPlate is that it's much easier for people to grasp the idea that half of a meal should consist of fruits and vegetables than it is for them to understand serving sizes for all the different kinds of foods they eat on a regular basis.

<u>Vitamins and fluid requirements</u>
Below are lists of wonderful sources of Vitamins A, C, and E:

- Vitamin A: Liver, Carrots, Sweet Potato/Yams, Butternut Squash, Mango, Cantaloupe, Apricots, Green leafy vegetables, Milk
- Vitamin C: Asparagus, Broccoli, Brussels Sprouts, Antelope, Kiwi, Papaya, Strawberries, Oranges, Red Pepper
- Vitamin E: Almonds, Hazelnuts, Spinach, Sweet Potatoes, Wheat Germ, Avocado, Peanuts, Sunflower Seeds, Various Vegetable Oils

Symptoms of dehydration include dry mouth, tongue and mucous membranes, decreased urination, sunken eyes, cheeks or abdomen, confusion, light-headedness, dizziness, disorientation, dry skin, fatigue, irritability, thirst, and weight loss, among others. It is recommended that humans consume a minimum 30 milliliters of fluid per kilogram body weight, daily.

Thus, the daily recommended fluid intake for a woman weighing 135 lbs is calculated as follows:
- Convert pounds to kilograms: 135 lbs x 0.454 kg/lb = 61.29 kg
- Daily recommended fluid intake: 61.29 kg x 30 mL/kg = 1838.7 mL

Below are lists of wonderful sources of calcium and vitamin D:
- Calcium: Dairy products, Tofu, Soybeans, Rhubarb, Salmon, Leafy-green vegetables, Oysters
- Vitamin D: Fortified milk and dairy products, Salmon, Herring, Sardines, Eggs, Some organ meats, Sunlight

**Note: Vitamin D aides the absorption of calcium but does not naturally occur in many foods. Sunlight is the best source of Vitamin D, though overexposure to the sun's rays may lead to cancer and other skin diseases. Brief exposure of the hands, face, and arms to the sun is generally sufficient.

Carbohydrate exchange system

The exchange system is one in which foods are grouped into six separate categories. Those categories are starches, such as pastas, rice, bread, and starchy vegetables, meat and meat substitutes, such as eggs, tofu, fish, and poultry, fruits, vegetables, milk, and fats. Another pseudo-category is that of "free foods." These foods contain small amounts of carbohydrates, and may, therefore, be consumed with greater freedom. Foods grouped within the same category will have similar amounts of fat, protein, and carbohydrates per serving. Therefore, one may "exchange" any food for another in the same category. The exchange system is particularly helpful in monitoring carbohydrates and is frequently used by patients with glycemic disorders, such as diabetes.

To calculate the number of grams of carbohydrates and protein contained in a meal that includes two starch exchanges, one fruit exchange, two vegetable exchanges, two meat exchanges, and one milk exchange, you need to know the exchange values per serving. Exchange values per serving are as follows:
- Starch: 15 g carbohydrates, 3 g protein
- Vegetable (non-starchy): 5 g carbohydrates, 2 g protein
- Fruit: 15 g carbohydrates, 0 g protein
- Milk: 12 g carbohydrates, 8 g protein
- Meat: 0 g carbohydrates, 7 g protein
- Fats: 0 g carbohydrates, 0 g protein

Therefore, to calculate grams of carbohydrates and proteins for two starch exchanges, one fruit exchange, two vegetable exchanges, two meat exchanges, and one milk exchange, you would do the following calculations:
- Grams carbohydrates = 2(15 g) + 15 g + 2(5 g) + 2(0 g) + 12 g = 67 g carbohydrates
- Grams protein = 2(3 g) + 0 g + 2(2 g) + 2(7 g) + 8 g = 32 g protein

HIPAA

HIPAA is the acronym for Health Insurance Portability and Accountability Act. This act became effective in 1996, and it is also known as the Kennedy-Kassebaum Act. The four main objectives of the act are to regulate computer-to-computer sharing of information (the "transaction standard"), provide universal identifiers for healthcare providers and healthcare plans, implement information security regulations, and establish a privacy rule. The privacy rule portion of HIPAA was instated in 2003, and it specifically deals with a patient's right to privacy in regards to his/her medical care. Upon an initial visit with a medical practitioner, all patients must receive and acknowledge receipt of a privacy notice. The patient's chart must always be handled with the utmost care and confidentiality, such that none other than the patient's care team has access to the information contained within his/her record. All records must be physically secured and/or password protected if electronically documented. Other than the medical team (to include treatment, payment, and healthcare operations personnel), only the patient and his/her designated representative are allowed access to the medical record. HIPAA does have additional disclosures which allow access to medical records in the interest of public health, law enforcement, research, government functions, etc.

Diseases

Diabetes

Diabetes is a disease in which the pancreas is not able to effectively regulate insulin production, and, therefore, the body's cells do not receive needed amounts of glucose. When an individual consumes carbohydrates, those carbohydrates are broken down into glucose, which immediately enters the bloodstream. In a correctly functioning body, the pancreas then produces insulin which aids in the cells' absorption of glucose. However, in patients with diabetes, the insulin production is either insufficient or dysfunctional and the glucose is unable to reach the cells. There are two long-term forms of diabetes. Type 1 Diabetes (more commonly known as juvenile-onset or insulin-dependent diabetes) occurs when the insulin-production system is permanently disabled. On the other hand, Type 2 Diabetes develops gradually and is often the result of poor diet and exercise habits. In this type, the cells no longer respond to insulin, and thus, the production of insulin begins to fail. If not properly treated and managed, diabetes can lead to many long-term health issues, including blindness, heart disease, stroke, foot and leg problems, and others. Diets designed specifically for diabetic patients should be formulated to promote healthy blood glucose, cholesterol, and blood pressure levels. Because diabetes is directly related to the body's ability to process, store, and utilize carbohydrates, it is important to monitor carbohydrate intake. While a well balanced diet that follows the guidelines set forth by the USDA is generally adequate for a patient with diabetes, many dietitians recommend an exchange diet, which allows the patient relative dietary freedom while still monitoring carbohydrate (sugar and starch) intake. Sugars may be substituted for starches in the exchange diet; however, doing so diminishes the nutritional value of the entire meal. Additionally, artificial sweeteners do not seem to have an effect on blood glucose. In addition to closely monitoring carbohydrate consumption, patients with diabetes should aim to eat a heart-healthy diet. Because of their increased risk for heart disease, avoiding trans and saturated fats as well as foods with high cholesterol content is advisable.

Kidney disease

Kidney disease affects the body's ability to process and eliminate waste and extraneous fluid from the body and blood stream. Dietary changes may help in the management of the disease. The most common dietary changes implemented in individuals with kidney disease include controlling the amount of protein and limiting phosphorus and sodium intake. Note the lists below which identify foods with high levels of protein, phosphorus, and sodium:

- Protein: Meat, Poultry, Seafood, Dairy Products, Eggs, Other Animal Products
- Phosphorus: Dairy Products, Dried beans, Dried Peas, Soft Drinks, Nuts, Peanut Butter
- Sodium: Table Salts, Processed Cheese, Canned/Prepared Meals, Pickled Foods, Fast Food, Cured Meats

Clients with kidney disease should also avoid multivitamins as the body has a difficult time breaking down some vitamins and minerals.

Cancer patients

Patients with cancer often suffer from a myriad of symptoms, which may affect their diets. Some common symptoms of cancer and side effects of treatment include fatigue, altered sense of taste and smell, nausea, vomiting, diarrhea, constipation, dry, sore mouth, and others. It is important that cancer patients receive a well-balanced diet, rich in vitamins and minerals. Additionally, because of their generally weakened immune system, patients with cancer should avoid raw, undercooked, and unpasteurized foods, all of which are more susceptible to bacteria. Frequently, clients with cancer will also be advised to follow a high-calorie diet, which provides greater energy to assist in combating fatigue. Employ strategies, such as adding additional sugar/sweetener, to enhance the flavors of the food and, in turn, make mealtime a more enjoyable experience.

Heart disease

Patients with cardiovascular disease may suffer from a variety of ailments, to include high blood pressure and cholesterol levels, high risk of stroke, heart attack, and more. Therefore, dietary modification is an effective way to prevent and treat patients with heart disease. Common recommendations include implementing a low-sodium (less than 2300 mg/day), low-cholesterol diet (less than 300 mg/day), eliminating trans fats by eliminating partially hydrogenated vegetable oils and fried foods, reducing sugar intake, and consuming only the calories needed to meet one's daily energy requirements. Additionally, it is advisable for patients at-risk or suffering from heart disease to increase their fruit and vegetable intake, maximizing vitamin, mineral, and antioxidant consumption, as well as to eat a diet high in fiber.

Iron deficiency

Iron deficiency is best combated by introducing or increasing iron-rich foods in one's diet. Additionally, consumption of Vitamin C rich foods will enhance the absorption of non-heme iron. Iron-rich foods include:

- Heme Iron Sources: Clams, Oysters, Shrimp, Organ Meats, Beef, Duck, Lamb
- Non-Heme Iron Sources: Fortified cereals, Soybeans, Squash, Pumpkin, Various Beans, Tomato Products, Prune Juice, Molasses

Iron deficiency can occur for a variety of reasons. Most commonly, individuals experiencing rapid growth (especially infants, children under five years of age, and pubescent females), pregnant women, and those who have lost large amounts of blood (through normal processes such as menstruation, infection or disease, or blood donation, for example) experience iron deficiency. Additionally, individuals who do not eat a healthy diet may also suffer from iron deficiency. Symptoms of an iron deficiency include tiredness/fatigue, slowed development, inability to regulate or maintain body temperature, and impaired immune system functioning, among others.

Pressure ulcers
Pressure ulcers, also known as pressure sores, bed sores, decubitus ulcers, and ischemic ulcers, occur when pressure is placed on one part of the body for too long, without repositioning. Essentially, layers of dermis gradually breakdown from unrelenting pressure to cause open wounds that vary in severity from a reddened area on the skin to an ulcer that has damaged muscle, bone, tendon, and other tissue. Causes of pressure sores include immobility, incontinence (moisture can contribute to tissue breakdown), malnourishment, diabetes and/or circulation problems. Therefore, these sores may be warning signs of malnourishment, in which a balanced, substantial diet needs to be introduced and/or other diseases, such as diabetes, in which other dietary action should also be taken.

Hemoglobin, hematocrit, and platelet blood values

Hemoglobin and hematocrit values, paired with red blood cell count, are particularly telling of iron-deficient anemia. If blood values are particularly low, an iron-rich diet and/or iron supplements should be considered. Additionally, consuming Vitamin C with non-heme iron sources will aid in the absorption of the iron. Healthy values for hematocrit and hemoglobin are as follows:
- Hematocrit: Male 40-54%, Female 37-47%, Children 31-41%
- Hemoglobin: Male 14-18 g/dL, Female 12-16 g/dL

Low platelet counts put patients at the risk of bleeding, as their bodies' ability to clot blood is impaired. Low platelets are often seen in individuals receiving a variety of therapeutic treatments, including radiation and chemotherapy. Diet should be adjusted to include extra fluids in order to avoid constipation. Additionally, increased protein intake and avoiding foods that may irritate the intestinal lining may be helpful to the client. A healthy blood platelet count is between 140,000-450,000 /mm^3.

Serum albumin, prealbumin, and transferrin levels

Albumin and transferrin levels are helpful data for dietitians in that they provide information about protein malnourishment. Additionally, albumin analysis may be helpful in determining whether a patient has kidney or liver disease. Moreover, transferrin binds iron and is essential to iron absorption. Thus, low transferrin levels may further indicate iron deficiency.

Acceptable blood levels are listed below:
- Serum Albumin - 3.4-5.4 g/dL
- Prealbumin - 18-45 mg/dL
- Transferrin - Male 130-315 mg/dL (age dependent), Female 140-340 mg/dL (age dependent)

*Note: Prealbumin is also referred to as transthyretin.

Apply Nutrition Data

Federal food, menu, and feeding schedule regulations

Federal regulations mandate that all facilities provide their clients with nourishing, palatable food that is presented as part of a well-balanced diet. Menus must satisfy total nutritional needs, be palatable and attractively presented. Additionally, a menu plan must be prepared in advance and followed. The food on the plan must be properly prepared and served at a healthy temperature. Moreover, the food and/or menu must be adapted for patients' individual needs. Patients who refuse food must be offered a substitute that has an equivalent nutritive value. Physician prescribed therapeutic diets must be followed. Finally, facilities must have at least three scheduled mealtimes, at regular intervals throughout the day. There may be no more than fourteen hours between a dinner meal and breakfast meal, except in the case where a nutritive snack is offered, in which the interval between those meals may be stretched to sixteen hours.

Assistive devices

Assisted devices are types of equipment that are adapted in order to make feeding easier for a client. Common assistive devices include a lip plate, weighted cups and utensils, rocker, curved, or t-shaped knives, various modified cups, including a lidded cup, pedestal cup, and Kennedy cup, utensils with large/wide handles, and various types of feeders which assist the patient in bringing food to the mouth (these are particularly useful for individuals with limited mobility of the upper extremities and/or those who are too weak to lift their hands to their mouths). Many of these devices are particularly useful for patients with tremors as well as those with impaired control of their hands.

Federal assistive device regulations

Federal regulations mandate that care facilities provide appropriate feeding assistive devices (lip plate, weighted utensils, cups, feeding devices, and others) and feeding staff where necessary. Paid staff who assist with feedings must work under the supervision of a licensed or registered nurse and must be trained. Training should be comprised of a minimum of eight hours of education on the following topics: feeding and hydration techniques and assistance, communication and behavioral response, safety procedures (to include the Heimlich maneuver), infection control, resident rights, and patient monitoring (so that an assistant may properly note and report any behavioral changes displayed by the client). These assistants are not allowed to feed patients with complicated feeding problems, to include those who have difficulty swallowing, have persistent/reoccurring aspiration of the lungs, and/or must be fed intravenously or through the use of a tube.

OBRA

OBRA is the acronym for Omnibus Budget Reconciliation Act (of 1987). This act greatly impacted long-term healthcare facilities, as it attempted to provide for the individual needs of patients. OBRA mandates that a facility provide the nutrition necessary for a patient to maintain an acceptable nutritional status, to include body weight as well as mineral and nutrient balance, except when a patient's health condition prevents it. Furthermore, OBRA ensures that patients receive a therapeutic and/or adapted diet when his/her condition warrants such modification. While this act protects many patients in long-term care facilities, it greatly affects daily food costs and preparation at long-term care facilities.

CMS

CMS is the acronym for Centers for Medicare and Medicaid Services. Medicare, a government health entity, provides funding for nutritional therapy for clients with renal disease as well as for those with diabetes. Medicare benefits include coverage for an initial assessment, nutrition counseling, provision of informational materials, and progress monitoring. In order to receive and continue Medicare benefits, doctors must prescribe therapeutic diets for patients. Additionally, to qualify for additional and/or extended benefits, a new therapeutic diet must be prescribed by the physician. CMS requires that care plans be developed for all beneficiaries.

Common cooking measurement equivalents

Common cooking volume, weight, and fluid measurement equivalents are as follows:
- 3 teaspoons = 1 tablespoon
- 16 tablespoons = 1 cup
- 8 ounces = 1 cup
- 2 cups = 1 pint
- 2 pints = 1 quart
- 4 quarts = 1 gallon
- 16 ounces = 1 pound

Special diet situations

Aging
Aging takes its toll on all of the body's systems, not least of which is the gastrointestinal system. Changes may occur in the mouth, which may include decreased production of saliva, changes in olfactory abilities, including the ability to taste, and changes in the teeth, gums, and palates. These changes may result in difficulties tasting, chewing, and swallowing food. Additionally, the gastrointestinal tract's ability to move food through via peristalsis may be impaired in the esophagus and stomach, which may further reduce one's ability to swallow, cause heartburn, cause heartburn, constipation, and other problems processing and metabolizing food. Other changes, including reduced blood flow to the gastrointestinal tract and liver may result in additional discomfort as the body's ability to process food is hindered.

Clear fluid diet
Clear fluid diets are typically ordered when a patient has some type of ailment or pending procedure of the digestive tract, to include colonoscopies, surgeries of the colon or rectum, difficulty swallowing, and so on. A clear fluid diet includes foods that one can see through including, but not limited to:
- Jello/Gelatin
- Various broths
- Fruit Juices
- Tea
- Carbonated beverages

- Sugar water
- Coconut water
- Water/Ice

Full fluid diet

A full fluid diet may be ordered when a patient has difficulty swallowing. Nearly any fluid may be included in this diet, including foods that melt at room temperature (such as ice cream). A full fluid diet may include, but is not limited to, the following foods:
- Strained soups
- Gelatin
- Pudding/Custard
- Milk
- Tea
- Carbonated beverages
- Fruit Juice
- Vegetable Juice
- Fine, hot cereals (Cream of Wheat)
- Ice cream/Sherbert
- Yogurt
- Coffee
- Watermelon
- Water/Ice

Pregnant women

Pregnant women should be encouraged to eat a healthy, balanced diet packed with fruits, vegetables, whole grains, protein, and dairy products. Typically, during her pregnancy, a healthy woman should consume between 200 and 400 more healthy calories per day. Depending on pre-pregnancy weight, caloric consumption may be more or less. Additionally, pregnant women have higher demands for vitamins and minerals, especially, folic acid, calcium, and iron. Pregnancy also demands large fluid stores in a woman's body, therefore pregnant woman should consume at least eight glasses (more with physical activity) of water per day. In addition to increasing nutrients, pregnant women should avoid some foods. Those foods include alcohol and some types of seafood with generally high mercury levels, namely, shark, swordfish, mackerel, or tilefish.

Pregnant women should consume additional folic acid and calcium in their diet. The following are foods that are rich in calcium and folate:
- Folic Acid: Enriched cereals, Enriched grains, Legumes, Black beans, Spinach, Asparagus, Green leafy vegetables, Lentils, Pinto Beans
- Calcium: Calcium-fortified juices, Calcium-fortified cereals, Dairy products, Green leafy vegetables, Almonds, Salmon, Tofu, Rhubarb, Beans

Therapeutic diet

A therapeutic diet is one that is specifically designed to meet a patient's needs. Therapeutic diets vary widely and may include orders to increase consumption of certain nutrients to presentation/adaptation of regularly served menu items. Generally, the facility diet manual will guide the physician in preparing his/her dietary orders. Though other healthcare team members are often consulted in regards to a patient's needs, a therapeutic diet may only be ordered or changed by a physician. Once that diet is ordered, a nutrition specialist and/or

- 14 -

dietary manager will generally oversee the manner in which the doctor's orders are implemented. Again, it is important to remember, that ONLY the physician may change, modify, or cancel a dietary order. Any questions regarding the order should be directed to the ordering physician and/or his staff dietitian.

Fluid restricted diet

A fluid restricted diet is most often ordered when a patient has a condition promoting fluid retention/edema or has renal disease. Fluid restricted diets limit the daily fluid intake. When estimating the total daily fluid intake, it is important to factor fluids consumed when taking medicine, eating meals and snacks, as well as those intravenously administered. It is also important to determine whether fluid restriction is taking into account the fluid content of a solid food. Patients on a fluid restricted diet must be closely monitored to ensure that they do not voluntarily consume greater quantities of fluid than is healthy.

High calorie, high protein diet

A high calorie, high protein diet is most often ordered for patients who have suffered a high degree of weight loss in a short period of time, those who were not able to eat anything by mouth over an extended period of time, and/or in failure to thrive cases. Physicians/nutritionists often recommend that cancer patients adhere to a high calorie, high protein diet in order to maintain their strength and combat fatigue during treatment. High calorie, high fat diets encourage consumption of whole dairy products, such as whole milk, ice cream, butter, and cream. Peanut butter, meats, nuts, avocado, and other similar foods may be great supplements to this diet.

Vegetarian diets

Vegetarians rely on plant sources as their primary source of food. There are three types of vegetarian diets. Vegan diets exclude all animal meats and products. Lacto-vegetarian diets allow consumption of plant and dairy products. The lacto-ovo-vegetarian diet incorporates dairy, egg, and plant products. Vegetarians often need to supplement their diet with alternative sources of calcium, protein, iron, and B12 vitamin. Tofu, soy, and nuts are helpful protein and calcium supplements. Enriched cereals and other grains are also helpful supplements to any of the above diets.

Low cholesterol diet

Low cholesterol diets are often used to help combat cardiovascular disease by controlling or reducing blood lipid and cholesterol levels. Typically, low cholesterol diets aim to limit cholesterol intake to 200-300 milligrams per day. By limiting or eliminating high cholesterol foods, one can easily lower the risk of heart disease. Cholesterol is only found in animal products. That is to say, cholesterol may be found in meats, poultry, seafood, eggs, and dairy products. Conversely, cholesterol is not present in plant products, even those with high fat content. Organ meats, especially liver, and eggs have particularly high cholesterol contents. To implement a low cholesterol diet, a client may limit animal product consumption and/or eat lean cuts of meat and low-fat dairy products. Additionally, adding more fruits, vegetables, and whole grains to the diet will help lower cholesterol.

Kosher diet

Practicing Orthodox Jews observe a kosher diet. That diet is derived from biblical texts in which certain foods are permitted and others are outlawed. Foods avoided by those on a kosher diet include meats such as pork and rabbit, seafood such as catfish, shellfish, and shrimp, certain types of foul, and any type of insect. Kosher regulations also include specific rules forbidding dairy products from coming in contact with meat, as well as specific regulations regarding cheese, wine, and some juices. Moreover, kosher foods must be prepared in a humane and painless manner, with a rabbi overseeing the animal slaughter. One should look for foods labeled kosher when preparing meals for a client on a kosher diet. Frequently, non-kosher foods are tainted by an ingredient derived from a non-kosher source.

Islamic clients

Similar to Orthodox Jews, Muslims practice certain dietary restrictions and observe a diet called Halal. Halal diets are very similar to kosher diets. Foods that are forbidden include pork, carnivorous and omnivorous animals, certain fowl, non-amphibious animals without external ears, and blood products. Muslims are allowed to eat fish-eating animals. Additionally, all permissible animal products must be properly slaughtered under the auspices of an expert. Halal diets also forbid any consumption of alcohol. Again, as with kosher diets, Halal diets are often exclusionary of prepared foods as ingredient sources may be unknown and/or improperly prepared.

Enteral feeding

Enteral feeding is any method of tube feeding where food is delivered directly to the stomach. There are several different types of tubes, and the type of tube may dictate the location of the device. For example, the tube may be inserted in various positions of the stomach or along other areas of the gastro-intestinal tract. Enteral tubes increase the risk of infection in patients as there is essentially an open line between one's environment and stomach. Therefore, feeding assistants should use the utmost care, to include hand washing and sanitization, utilizing sanitized equipment, properly flushing and caring for the tube, and following any procedures specific to the patient, when assisting with tube feedings. Enteral tubes are most often used in patients who have lost their ability to swallow and/or have diminished peristalsis.

Parenteral feeding

Parenteral feeding is a method of feeding in which nutrients are delivered directly to the blood stream through the use of a catheter. Parenteral feeding completely bypasses the digestive system and is frequently used in patients who have had part of their digestive system removed or are having severe problems digesting foods and are lacking essential nutrients. Like patients who receive enteral feedings, those receiving parenteral feedings are highly susceptible to infection, and therefore, feedings must be handled with the utmost of care by the patient and caregivers. Additionally, the patient's environment should be kept extremely clean. The nutrients delivered parenterally are combined to create a specific formula. Various drugs may affect the formulas and should be carefully added to patient's regimen.

Long-term care setting care plan

In a long-term care setting, a care plan is developed after the initial assessment. The initial assessment must be completed within fourteen days of patient admittance. Then, the care plan is developed to ensure that the client's needs are met. This care plan includes any special dietary orders, including prescription of a therapeutic diet, and it must be completed within seven days of the completion of the initial assessment. Thus, within 21 days of

- 16 -

admittance to a long-term care facility, every patient should have a personalized care plan. Assuming that there are no changes in a patient's health, the care plan must be updated quarterly. Otherwise, the care plan should be revisited with every significant change in the patient's health.

There are some ways in which the supporting staff at a long-term healthcare facility may learn about customer meal preferences and habits. The following methods may give insight to a client's meal preferences and habits:
- Observe the patient at mealtime. Note what is eaten, what is left untouched, and how much an individual consumes.
- Interview customers in regards to meal satisfaction. This may be done formally or informally. Interviews may be presented orally or written and/or comment cards may be left for clients.
- Calculate plate waste. Note if there is a pattern and/or if there is a greater percentage of certain items that are left uneaten in comparison to other menu items.
- Randomly test plates for food temperature and note presentation of food.
- Form an advisory council of residents, staff, and patient family members to provide feedback and offer suggestions to improve menu options.

Diet liberalization

A liberalized diet is one in which the patient is given a greater level of freedom in regards to his/her diet. That is not to say, however, that a liberalized diet ignores therapeutic dietary orders. Rather, by allowing dietary liberalization, patients exercise their right and ability to make decisions in regards to their menu. That decision making should be both preceded and followed by dietary counseling. The thinking behind this method stems from the idea that most clients are malnourished and must first get healthy before focusing on dietary restrictions. The freedom of choice encourages clients to eat rather than to feel subjected to another's menu and plan. Counseling then begins to shape the menu choices that clients continue to make. Both the benefits of eating healthy and the consequences of eating poorly should be emphasized. In some cases, adjunct pharmacotherapy may need to be implemented to ensure overall health. A liberalized diet may also simplify food preparation for an institution, in that it means fewer specialized diets. It is always important to remember, however, that the client's health is paramount to operational simplicity.

Eating and food disorders

Anorexia nervosa
Anorexia nervosa is a psychiatric disorder in which patients refuse to eat in order to achieve a certain body-image. Though individuals suffering from anorexia may literally be starving, the individual most often sees himself/herself as overweight. Anorexia nervosa causes extreme malnourishment and may present via symptoms such as weight loss, sunken eyes, protruding skeletal structure, amenorrhea, constipation, fatigue, low energy, downy hair on the face and neck, and other symptoms. Therapy focusing on behavior modification is essential to recovery from anorexia. Primary dietary concerns are to address malnourishment and introduce healthy eating habits. The diet gradually increases caloric consumption and may aim for more than three meals per day.

Bulimia nervosa
Bulimia is an eating disorder characterized by binging and purging. Purging may be achieved by vomiting or taking laxatives. Bulimia drains the body of all nutrients and electrolytes and causes various digestive tract problems resulting from the constant strain on the system from purging. Bulimia further affects nearly every body system including the cardiac, endocrine, and nervous systems. As with anorexia, behavioral therapy is the recommended treatment. Healthy dietary habits should be introduced and malnourishment immediately addressed. A diet that gradually increases caloric consumption should be prescribed.

Celiac disease
Celiac disease attacks the small intestine and creates sensitivity to gluten. Gluten is found in wheat, barley, and rye products. Additionally, many products are produced in factories that also manufacture gluten-containing products. Thus, individuals with celiac disease must search for "gluten-free" products. "Gluten-free" products may include any product that does not have the opportunity to come in contact with gluten and extends beyond pastas, breads, and flours. Dietary substitutions for foods containing gluten include soy, rice, potato, nuts, legumes, tapioca, corn, flax seed, and buckwheat.
Note: Many vitamins, supplements, and pharmaceuticals also contain gluten. Advise clients to check with their pharmacist before taking any medicines.

Lactose intolerance
Lactose is the primary sugar found in milk products. An individual who exhibits lactose intolerance lacks the enzyme that breaks down the lactose to an easily digestible form. Individuals who are lactose intolerant should avoid many dairy products but should still strive to meet daily calcium recommendations. Calcium may be garnered through other sources, such as by consuming dark, green vegetables, soy, tofu, salmon, sardines, beans, and oranges. Some individuals are able to tolerate yogurt with live bacteria cultures as the bacteria has the enzyme necessary to breakdown the lactose.
Note: Many non-dairy, processed foods may also contain lactose, which was added during the preparation process. Additionally, vitamins, supplements, and prescription drugs may also contain lactose.

Dysphagia
Patients suffering from dysphagia, or difficulty swallowing, may display a variety of symptoms. Those symptoms include:
- Coughing when eating
- Choking when eating
- Unexplained or rapid weight loss
- Unexplained change in dietary habits
- Change in voice or speech patterns
- Drooling
- Dehydration
- Refusal to eat
- Food aversions
- Recurrent pneumonia

Dysphagia, or difficulty swallowing, can drastically change one's quality of life, as it affects one's ability to eat, speak, and perform other similar tasks. When a patient is diagnosed with dysphagia, he or she often begins working with a speech therapist. Some commonly used therapies for an individual with dysphagia include modifying texture of diet as well as physical exercises. Those exercises include posture modification to aid in swallowing, exercises performed while swallowing, as well as exercising the muscles in the mouth and neck while not eating. *Note: Use of enteral feedings may be necessary for patients with dysphagia.

Food and Nutrition Services

Provide Food Services

Serving and portion size

Though often used interchangeably, portion size and serving size are not necessarily equivalent amounts of food. Portion size is the amount of food that one serves up and consumes. Thus, portion size may vary from person to person. On the contrary, serving size refers to the amount of food for which the nutritional values refer. A serving size may or may not match the recommended portion size of a food. For example, if one were to compare the serving size of various cereals he might find that one brand recommends a serving size of three-quarters of a cup whereas another brand may recommend a serving size of one cup. The nutritional values reflect the fat, calorie, and vitamin content of one serving.

<u>American Dietetic Association serving sizes</u>
The American Dietetic Association recommends modest portion sizes, equivalent to the below serving sizes:
- Meat, 3 ounces
- Margarine, 1 teaspoon
- Pasta, 1 cup
- Cheese, 1 ½ ounces
- Bread, 1 slice or 1 ounce
- Bagel, ½ medium
- Peanut butter, 2 tablespoons
- Milk, 1 cup
- Vegetables, ½ cup

<u>Common exchange diet portions</u>
Exchange diets are specifically formulated to direct patients with diabetes to eat a healthy diet that regulates carbohydrate intake. Below are the portions equivalent to one exchange:
- Bread, 1 ounce
- Cooked pastas, cereals, grains, ½ cup
- Meat (cooked), 1 ounce
- Vegetables (raw), 1 cup
- Vegetables (cooked), ½ cup
- Vegetables (juiced), ½ cup
- Milk, 1 cup
- Fats, 1 teaspoon

Likert Scale

The Likert Scale is a rating system in which people respond by assigning a number or word to their degree of satisfaction with the object in question. This scale is a helpful survey tool as it neither influences client response nor does it make it difficult for a client to respond. Thus, a dietary manager may use this scale when surveying clients in regards to food service. A sample question is as follows:

- Rate the attractiveness of served plates.
  Excellent   Good   Average   Needs Improvement   Poor

Or, it may be phrased as:

- On a scale of 1 to 5, with one being poor and five being excellent, rate the attractiveness of served plates.

Calculating percentage in survey results

In order to calculate percentage, one must first count the total number of survey respondents. Then, count how many people chose each response. Finally, divide the number people choosing each response by the number of respondents and repeat this procedure for each response. See the example below for sample calculations.

Ninety-eight people responded to a food service survey. When asked to rate the attractiveness of served plates, 63 people responded with "Excellent;" 22 with "Good;" 7 with "Average;" 5 with "Needs Improvement;" and 1 with "Poor." Show a summary of the ratings, in percentages:

- Excellent: (63/98) x 100 = 64.3%
- Good: (22/98) x 100 = 22.4%
- Average: (7/98) x 100 = 7.1%
- Needs Improvement: (5/98) x 100 = 5.1%
- Poor: (1/98) x 100 = 1.0 %

Plate waste

Plate waste is the amount of food left uneaten on a plate by a client. Waste is estimated by comparing the portion size to the amount of food remaining on the plate. It is important to note plate waste as it is a good indicator of client preferences. If a served menu item consistently results in a large amount of plate waste, it is likely that the clients do not prefer that item. Additionally, if a menu item is often well received but on one occasion results in an abnormally large plate waste, the food may not have been properly prepared, served, and/or was not the correct temperature. On the other hand, if a menu item does not consistently result in plate waste that is a good indicator that the menu item is well received by the institution's clients.

Tray-line system

A tray-line system is a streamlined method of preparing trays for clients. This system operates in an assembly-line fashion in which trays are passed (either manually or by conveyor belt) from one food service worker to another. In the instances where clients are given menu options, foods are most often grouped according to where they fall on the menu. As the trays are passed, food service workers prepare trays using the selected menu items for each individual. It is important that tray-line employees ensure that menu selections match the finished tray and that trays are handled quickly and efficiently. Employee distractions may result in a health risk to clients as delayed delivery of food compromises the temperature of the prepared items.

The typical steps of a healthcare facility tray-line are as follows:
1. Distribute menus to patients. Most facilities offer some level of patient choice in regards to their meals. Even limited menus are preferable to those with no choice.
2. Collect patient menu selections.
3. If using electronic equipment to convey menu selections, the patients' selections must be entered into the system. Otherwise, menus are sorted, generally by room and ward and delivered to the kitchen.
4. Ensure menus are sorted by ward. Prepare to assemble trays.
5. Send ticket on tray down the tray-line for assembly.
6. Trays are collected according to ward, and placed on transporter.
7. Trays are delivered to ward.
8. Nurses, aides, or other staff members deliver patient trays to rooms. Prompt delivery is essential to preserving food quality.

There are many tools and procedures available to ensure proper temperature control of food originating at a tray-line. For example, an institution may choose to deliver food on an insulated tray or utilizing dinnerware that contain warming plates. Additionally, many tray transporters have temperature controlling properties, whether those consist of insulation or continuous heat. Finally, quick tray assembly and prompt delivery of the food is paramount. Not only does quick delivery promote correct temperature at delivery but it also enhances the attractiveness of the plate as foods are not allowed the opportunity to "wilt."

A tray-line efficiency study is a method of evaluating the effectiveness, quickness, and organization of a tray-line. A study can be carried out via a variety of methods. One such method is to calculate the number of trays per minute leaving the tray-line. Another method is to intercept a sample of the trays between assembly and delivery and to calculate the rate of accuracy of prepared trays compared to selected menu items. Additionally, randomly testing trays between assembly and delivery for proper food temperature is another method of determining tray-line efficiency. A tray-line efficiency study is important in that it allows a dietary manager to see a greater picture of what is happening on the tray-line. If food is being served cold, perhaps the assembly is taking too long. If a menu item is not being properly served, there may be an issue with a tray-line employee. Furthermore, tray-line efficiency studies may be helpful in justifying additional hires of food service employees.

A trays per minute calculation is most often included in a tray-line efficiency study. To calculate trays per minute, one must first record the amount of time it takes to assemble trays. Do this by timing from the beginning of tray assembly until the last tray leaves the tray-line. Measure the time in minutes. Next, count the number of trays that left the line during the recorded time. Now, divide the number of trays assembled by the number of recorded minutes. So, if a tray-line was operating for thirty minutes and ninety trays were assembled, one would calculate the trays per minute by using the following equation:
- (Trays assembled)/ (Minutes of assembly) = Trays per minute
- (90 trays)/ (30 minutes) = 3 trays per minute

Tray-line accuracy is used to estimate the number of errors occurring during tray-line assembly. Accuracy rates are important determinants of tray-line efficiency. Fewer tray errors mean greater efficiency. To calculate tray-line accuracy, select a random sampling of trays. A greater sample size will produce more accurate data; however, one should be mindful of time when performing a tray-line accuracy survey. Delaying trays for the sake of the study is unacceptable. Using the tray tickets, count the total number of items for each tray, and add those tray totals together. Next, compare the tray ticket to the actual tray. Count the number of errors. Errors could include missing items, serving an item incorrectly, and/or inclusion of unordered items. Then, divide the total number of errors by the total number of ordered tray-line items. The product will equal the percent error. The smaller the error, the greater the tray-line accuracy.

An example follows:
- Tray 1 (T1): 10 items, 1 error; T2: 12 items, 0 errors; T3: 11 items, 2 errors; T4: 12 items, 3 errors
- Total number of errors: 6
- Total number of items: 45
- Percent error: [(6 errors)/ (45 items)] x 100 = 13%, Thus, the tray is accurate 87% of the time.

Buffet and family-style service

Buffet is the type of service in which all menu items are displayed buffet style, usually on temperature regulated tables conducive to self-service. Clients are able to browse the items and select the items that they would like to consume. Generally buffets include a wide-range of menu options. Foods are typically grouped according to temperature and compatibility. Additionally, buffets give clients the freedom to choose their own portion sizes. Family-style dinner service is such that customers sitting at a table pass serving dishes to one another. Each person is able to choose the food he/she is interested in as well as the portion. Menu options are limited to a specific meal.

Cafeteria service

Cafeteria service is a method of food service in which customers may select from a wide variety of items to assemble an individual meal. There are a various types of cafeteria models. Some arrangements promote self-service while others require a food service worker to serve the client. Some cafeterias are arranged such that a client must follow a line and select foods as he/she moves along. Conversely, many cafeterias have adopted a "scramble system" in which customers may float from station to station to choose menu items. The advantage of this system is that a client does not have to wait in line unnecessarily, and therefore, scramble systems generally promote faster food service.

Wait-service and self-service

Wait-service refers to the type of food service wherein wait staff bring prepared plates to the tables and present the plates to clients. Depending upon the size of the staff and institutional procedures, the roles and responsibilities of wait staff vary. This type of service is labor intensive and is not often utilized at institutions because of the high labor costs. On the other hand, self-service is when a client serves him/herself. This method is effective in minimizing costs as food service staff may be kept at a minimum. It does, however, promote the greatest freedom of dietary choice which can undermine the purpose of therapeutic diets.

Cycle menu

A cycle menu is one where different menus are planned for each day over a specified period of time. At the end of that period, the entire cycle menu is repeated. A cycle may take as few as three to four days or may be as long as a couple of months. When used correctly, a cycle menu allows food service personnel to more effectively order food and prepare meals. Because the overall menu is repeated, the kitchen staff may more easily anticipate food, time, and labor needs. Additionally, clients know what to expect of the menu and may look forward to certain meals.

A cycle menu runs the risk of becoming too repetitive, which may result in clients becoming bored with the menu. For this reason, longer cycles are preferable to shorter ones. Additionally, when utilizing a cycle menu, it is advisable to avoid matching menu items to certain days of the week. For example, offering pasta on Monday, chicken on Tuesday, and so on, every week, only emphasizes the repetitive nature of the menu. If, instead, one matches menu items to Day 1, Day 2, and so on, and if the cycle is not repeated every seven days, the menu will appear to be much less repetitive to many clients.

Making dining appealing

Simple touches can make dining much more attractive to clients. Some of those touches include:
- Fill the plate with a variety of color. Pair brightly colored fruits and vegetables with meats, poultry, and fish.
- Use fresh herbs as garnish. Drizzle or pipe sauces on foods rather than pouring or ladling sauces.
- Consider purchasing two coordinating sets of tableware. A change in plate color may make food pop. Additionally, tables may be set with a combination of the sets.
- Add flowers to the table. Use a variety of colored table linens. Ensure linens are clean and without stains.
- Serve food quickly to prevent "wilting" of meats, fruits, and vegetables or "cooking" of items left on heat plates.
- Do not overcook food. Again, the appearance of dried or "wilted" food is unappetizing.
- Make the tables and menu items easily available to everyone. Have adequate space for wheelchairs and adaptive equipment.

Individuals will naturally be more excited to eat when the dining facility and food presented look appealing. Appetizing presentation is particularly important in long-term care facilities where many patients are often suffering from some type of vitamin/mineral deficiency, malnourishment, and depression. Careful and colorful arrangement of food on a plate may entice customers to not only eat but also to try all of the menu items. Thus, if menus are planned correctly, clients have a greater chance of consuming a well-balanced meal. Mealtime is also the perfect time to meet others and pry patients away from the isolation of their rooms. Thus, a pleasurable dining experience will serve patients on a physical, emotional, and social level.

Food acceptance survey

A food acceptance survey assists a dietary manager in soliciting the opinions of his/her customer. This survey should include questions regarding food temperature, tastes, attractiveness, portion size, and other factors. Feedback from the survey should be addressed by the dietary staff, and it is advisable to form an advisory panel of staff, customers, and, in the case of a long-term care facility, patient families, that follows up the survey with discussion of the results as well as problem-solving brainstorms. When designing a food acceptance survey, it is important to be as specific as possible without leading clients. Vague questions will solicit vague answers which may cause frustration when attempting to improve/revise current service. Dissatisfaction expressed via the survey should be directly addressed by investigating alternative cooking and serving methods, changing menu items, utilizing different ingredients, performing tray-line efficiency studies, etc.

Federal regulations regarding posted menus

Federal regulations mandate that menus not only be followed, but that they are prepared in advance and in accordance to the recommendations of the Food and Nutrition Board of the National Research Council, National Academy of Sciences. Deviation from the posted menu is only allowed in the cases where a client refuses food. In such cases, a menu substitute may be offered as long as it has similar nutritional value to the posted menu item. In addition to federal regulations regarding posted menus, facilities must also follow any regulations mandated by the state in which the facility operates. As law is continuously evolving, it is important to review state and federal law regularly to ensure compliance.

Special nourishments

Special nourishments are commonly called:
- Nutritional supplements
- Medical food
- Food for special diets
- Oral supplements
- Liquid meals
- Medical supplements

Special nourishments may be orally, enterally or parenterally consumed. The name of the nourishment may or may not reflect the manner in which it is administered to the patient.

Special nourishments are most often administered to patients who are malnourished, lose at least five percent of body weight in a month's time, are unable to consume solid or pureed diets, have a specific medical condition that makes it difficult for the individual to swallow, digest, or process food, or those with severely progressed dementia. The decision to prescribe special nourishments should be made by an interdisciplinary team that takes into account a patient's total wellness—physical, emotional, and psychological-- as well as all of the patient's limitations. Patient conditions may digress such that he or she moves from a regular, balanced diet, to a pureed diet, to enteral feedings, and then, parenteral feedings. Additionally, a patient may receive supplemental nourishment even when able to consume food orally.

Supplements

Appropriate supplemental products
The appropriateness of a supplemental product relies on several factors. Those factors include:
- Ability of the supplement to meet all of the nutritional needs. Supplemental nourishment may need to provide a boost of certain nutrients, minerals, or elements of food. Alternatively, special nourishment may need to provide total nourishment for a client.
- Compatibility with any dietary restrictions brought about by allergy or disease.
- Cost and availability of product.
- Safety of product from production to intake.
- Life of product and suspected length of time nourishment will be needed.

Proper supplement preparation
When preparing supplements, great care must be taken to ensure patient health. Proper sanitation (to include hand washing, utilizing sanitized cooking/preparation equipment, and properly cleansing feeding devices) is paramount. Because many patients receiving supplemental nourishment are receiving the food via a tube or IV and because those patients are often already weak, they are at greater risk of infection. Additionally, care should be taken to ensure that the nourishment conforms to the prescribed diet. Because each client's supplement should be prepared specifically for him/her, it is essential to check the supplement against the individual's therapeutic diet.

Patients not receiving their supplements
Patient supplements are not optional; rather, they are a necessity and mandated by law. Therefore, it is imperative that supplements be passed to patients properly and on schedule. In the event that patients do not receive their prescribed supplements, the nursing staff must be held accountable. Thus, the shift charge nurse as well as the director of nursing should be notified. Additionally, the staff dietitian and attending physician all need to be made aware of the problem. The responsible party should be counseled and the incident documented. In the event of continued problems, it may be prudent to terminate the staff member.

Supplemental nourishment refusal
If a patient refuses supplemental nourishment, it is important to discuss his/her decision with the entire care team. Coordinate an opportunity for the care team to meet with the patient as well as the patient's family. Explain why the supplement was prescribed and how it may help the patient. Discuss alternative supplement options. If the patient and/or his family still refuse supplemental nourishment, document. It is important to note in the patient's chart who was at the meeting, what was discussed, as well as the patient's persistence to refuse supplemental nourishment. It is also advisable to have the patient and/or his family sign a document acknowledging the risks of refusing supplements and noting that such refusal was an informed, voluntary decision.

CQI

CQI is the acronym for Continuous Quality Improvement. CQI is any method used that monitors and strives for continuous improvement of departmental procedures. CQI is meant to be proactive, not reactive. Most CQI contain some variation on the following procedures:

- Describe objectives of plan and identify areas needing improvement
- Brainstorm methods to meet objectives and take corrective action where needed
- Develop methods into a standard operational plan
- Establish quality standards as benchmarks to assess effectiveness of plan
- Communicate SOP, quality standards, and goals to employees
- Implement plan
- Monitor operational reality of plan and assess improvement
- Accumulate and evaluate data measuring the success of the plan
- Revise SOP as necessary

Continuous Quality Improvement (CQI) procedures are unique to each facility and/or organization. Each facility has its strengths and weaknesses, and those must be identified and addressed in the facility's individual CQI. The operational manual of the facility should guide an interdisciplinary team in formulating and/or revising any CQI procedures. Moreover, each facility must establish specific quality standards for that particular facility. Those standards must guide the work output of all employees. When a quality standard fails to be met, employees should be counseled. Continual failure to meet quality standard may result in termination of an employee or revision of the standard.

Continuous Quality Improvement procedures should be utilized in every aspect of business and care. This extends from food preparation to delivery, menu and recipe development to the performance of employees and beyond. CQI that are communicated to all employees serve to improve the overall efficiency, morale, and product output of a facility. When employees know what is expected of them and their products, those individuals can work towards specific goals and benchmarks. CQI not only allows employees to do this, but they also ensure customer health and satisfaction as well as establish an evaluation system.

Audits

An audit is a method of evaluating an organization's compliance to and implementation of established operating procedures, regulations, and industry standards. Audits are typically performed by outside agencies, though organizations can impose a self-audit. Self-audits are great tools for evaluation and to ensure the organization is operating at the highest standards, thus avoiding penalties from regulating agencies when it comes time for their audit of the organization. Scheduling periodic self-audits also ensures that an organization continually complies with procedures, standards, and regulations, and allows problem areas to be addressed quickly. Food service audits will help to ensure healthy food preparation, prompt delivery of food items, menu compliance, and all other aspects of the industry. Audits easily identify problem areas which then may be addressed via CQI processes.

Self-audits may be difficult to carry out, as the "inspector" must objectively examine all the areas to be evaluated. However, the benefits of a self-audit far outweigh the disadvantages. To perform a self-audit, it is advisable to compile an evaluation list, taking industry, regulating agency, and facility standards into account. For example, in a healthcare facility, it is important to include standards put forth by the facility manual, those imposed by the health department, as well as regulations mandated by federal law/programs, such as Medicare/Medicaid. The evaluation list should avoid generic benchmarks; rather, specific standards should be listed. So, instead of evaluating plate presentation, standards such as appearance of food, temperature of food, cleanliness of plate, etc, may be scrutinized. Finally, categorize the evaluation list to streamline the process. Once a self-audit is carried out, establish a corrective plan of action for all problem areas.

Food cost and quality

While cost often reflects food quality, cost and quality are not always synonymous. Food producers and manufacturers employ a variety of methods for determining cost. It may be dependent upon the quality of food, extent of packaging, expense of transportation, or amount of food purchased at once. It is always important to evaluate the quality of food prior to purchasing. Additionally, a food acceptance survey may be used as a tool for selecting brands based upon client desires. However, be careful to include only affordable brands on the food acceptance survey.

Diet and menu modification

There are many available resources to aid in menu modification. Those resources include:
- Facility Dietary Manual. This should be the primary resources when modifying a diet as it will list commonly used substitutions, facility standards and limitations.
- American Dietetic Association
- American Heart Association
- American Diabetes Association
- American Cancer Society
- National Institutes of Health
- Advocate organizations for specific diseases
- Books addressing specific topics, i.e., aging, disease, etc.

Menu modifications may be necessary for a variety of reasons. Some of those reasons may include:
- Physical limitations of the client, for example, an inability to properly chew and swallow food
- Limitations imposed by a disease and/or gastrointestinal intolerance for or allergy to specific foods
- Change in health status, to include weight gain or loss or nutrient deficiency
- Preparation or recovery from a surgery, illness, or gastrointestinal irritation
- Dementia which impairs ability to feed oneself or memory to do so
- Taste aversions and refusal to eat certain foods
- Religious or ethnic restrictions

Recommendations from speech therapists

Speech therapists are trained to evaluate swallowing and feeding disorders as well as speech disorders. Because feeding and swallowing involve the tongue, mouth, pharynx, larynx, and esophagus (all of which influence one's ability to speak), speech therapists are proficient at working with clients to improve swallowing ability. Therapy is meant to improve dysphagia (difficulty swallowing) by determining the precise mechanism that is hindered or failing. Speech therapists may recommend the use of enteral feeding products either as a means of nourishing a client during therapy, with a goal of tube removal or may recommend enteral feedings when therapy does not remedy the dysphagia.

Finger-foods

As patients age and/or their health declines, they may adopt various adaptations in order to preserve their quality of life. One such adaptation is to eat using one's fingers versus utensils. A patient may do this because he or she lacks strength in the upper extremities and/or because the patient's coordination has deteriorated. In such cases, menu modification may be necessary. Small dietary modifications, such as serving chicken strips versus whole chicken breasts, crudités in place of salad, and cookies or cupcakes in lieu of cakes may be helpful. Additionally, liquid items, such as soups and ice cream, may be served in an easily held cup. Slight menu modifications such as these allow the patient to maintain his/her quality of life and dignity. However, it is important that the patient be frequently monitored for additional changes so that he or she receives adequate nourishment.

Provide Nutritional Information

Effective nutritional education

The effectiveness of nutritional education is largely dependent upon the delivery of that information. First, consider the audience—will information be delivered to children, adults, or the elderly? Does the individual have the cognitive ability to digest the information? Consider the attention span and energy level of the individual and attempt to counsel him/her during his/her most alert part of the day. Next, prepare the information in a manner suitable to the individual's learning style. Always leave notes and/or a pamphlet of information behind. Counsel the individual in regards to his/her dietary limitations, necessary changes, deficiencies, etc. Provide tools and motivation for the individual to make the necessary changes. Make suggestions to enhance long-term outcomes. It is important that emphasis be placed on the need for change. If the client does not understand the need for dietary change, the nutritional education will be for naught.

Nutritional education resources

There are many resources available to individuals wishing to change their eating habits. Resources are available in the community and virtually. Some of those resources include:
- Virtual Resources - Mypyramid.gov, American Heart Association website, American Cancer Society website, American Diabetes Association website, American Dietetics Association website, USDA website
- Community Resources - Home healthcare agencies, local nursing associations, local dietary associations, Meals on Wheels, senior services/centers

Portion size education

When educating a client in regards to portion size, it is helpful to provide everyday comparisons, or models, for portion size. This allows a client to more adequately "eyeball" the correct portion size. Some common comparison models are as follows:
- Meat, 1 oz. = Matchbox
- Meat, poultry, 3 oz. (typical serving size) = Deck of cards or palm of hand
- Cheese, 1 oz = 4 dice
- Potato, medium = Computer mouse
- Peanut butter, 2 Tbsp = Ping pong or golf ball
- Pasta, ice cream, ½ cup = Tennis ball or a cupped hand
- Bagel = Hockey puck
- Fruits/Vegetables = Baseball
- Pancake/Waffle = CD
- Fish, 3 oz. = Checkbook

Determining interest in learning

There are many cues that may indicate an individual's interest to learn new material. Some of those are evident by body language. An individual who looks eager often is. Eagerness may be indicated by attention to the speaker/counselor, interest in taking notes, making eye contact, asking questions, welcoming the individual, and other similar cues. On the other hand, someone with crossed arms, avoiding eye contact, appearing tired or uninterested, and/or changing the subject may not be ready to discuss any topic, let alone a topic regarding nutritional education. Additionally, ask the individual if he or she is motivated to make dietary changes. If the client responds positively, then begin the conversation. Finally, note whether the client is inquisitive either verbally or non-verbally.

Discerning understanding

Patient understanding is paramount to proper treatment and therapy. It is important, therefore, to determine whether an individual understands received counseling and nutritional education. Evaluate the level of a patient's understanding by asking the patient questions about topics discussed. Additionally, ask the patient if he or she can and will recap the discussion and/or action plan set forth. Moreover, the educator may also ask if the patient has any questions and what those questions are. It is appropriate to lead the patient to ask specific questions that will direct the discussion to key points of the educational session.
*Note: It is always appropriate and prudent to leave printed educational materials for further review and for patient reference.

Selective menus

Selective menus are designed to aid patients in healthy food choices. These particular menus allow patients a choice of menu items that when combined provide a well-balanced meal. By allowing patients to choose menu items, the facility is essentially granting greater patient autonomy. Additionally, patients consistently see healthy menus, comprised of items that, taken in whole, make a well-balanced meal. Therefore, patients learn through the use of a directed example how to pair menu items to create healthy meals. Not only are the patients learning how to create a well-balanced meal, but they are also being directed towards healthy foods and away from high-fat, high-sugar sources. Additionally, proper portion sizes of the menu items will further enforce healthy eating habits.

Food substitutions for patient preferences

Patient preference is important to ensuring consumption of a well-balanced meal. Selective menus are helpful in melding both patient preference and providing an equal distribution of vitamins and minerals. When substituting menu items, it is important that menu items of similar or equal nutritional value are substituted. Typically, fruits and vegetables whose meats are of similar color or structure may be substituted for each other. Often times, poultry may be substituted for other meats. In some cases, nutritional supplements may need to be administered to patients who consistently refuse to eat certain types of food groups. The primary objective, in all cases, is to provide the patient with a well-balanced diet.

Helpful learning tools

Various materials may be helpful in imparting nutritional education to clients. The type of materials may be determined by age, ailment afflicting patients, and type of information to be conveyed to the patients. Some helpful materials are listed below:
- Pamphlets and brochures recapping information. Be sure to have large-print, Braille, and picture pamphlets handy.
- Food models and portion size comparison models, including a deck of cards, balls of various sizes (tennis, ping pong, golf ball, etc), dice, matchbooks, and modeling with client's hand.
- Pictures and graphics of plates representing well-balanced meals, personalized food plan.
- Exchange diet equivalents.
- Diagram explaining how to read/dissect nutritional facts labeling information.
- Computer-generated aging programs, if available.

Dietary counseling structure

It is important that dietary counseling/education be methodically prepared and presented. In order to do so, the client's health and dietary needs are first assessed by the dietary manager and the patient's care team. After the assessment, a plan with future dietary changes and goals must be developed and followed. In order for the plan to be implemented, the developed plan must be realistic in its expectations. Finally, ongoing evaluations must be performed in order to ensure that the needs found by the assessment are, in fact, being addressed by the developed plan and implemented by the patient and care team. An evaluation of the plan may be used to revise dietary goals and plan expectations.

Written materials

Written materials are essential elements of patient education as they serve as a source of reference outside of dietary counseling sessions. Patients with impaired memory, who experience difficulty concentrating, and/or are suffering from fatigue may rely on written materials to guide their nutritional choices. The most effective written materials are printed in an easy to read font, that is both stylistically simplistic and of adequate size. Capitalization and punctuation should be properly utilized. Additionally, the materials should be kept as simple as possible, minimizing the use of complex sentences, large words, vocabulary consisting of medical and/or scientific jargon, and inclusion of excessive information. Spacing between lines and paragraphs should be such that the information may be easily read. Graphics and/or diagrams may be used to help explain topics, though excessive use of pictures may detract from the message being conveyed.

Customization

It is crucial that nutritional counseling be tailored to the individual, as each person has specific and unique needs. Even among individuals prescribed the same diets, it is imperative that each person receive specialized and individual counseling. Elements of counseling should include information about the patient's nutritional needs and restrictions, which should be personalized based upon the individual's taste preferences, regional recipes, and religious and/or cultural observances. Additionally, learning materials, including visual aids, videos, food portion models, and other similar tools should also be tailored to the individual being counseled. An individual with impaired vision, for example, should be provided large print reading materials and/or audio notes. Finally, take into account any adaptive equipment that an individual may use during mealtime. The adaptive equipment may influence the individual's willingness and ability to eat certain items. Patients may also need to be taught how to effectively utilize adaptive equipment.

Counseling techniques

Various counseling techniques may be used to convey nutritional information, implement a healthy program, and set goals for future progress. Some of the following techniques may be helpful:
- Assess whether the patient is ready and motivated to make behavior changes and modification. If so, proceed with nutritional counseling. If not, it is imperative that the counselor impress upon the client the need for change. If the individual is not willing to make changes, further counseling will be for naught.
- Help the client set realistic goals. If the client feels empowered, he or she is more apt to reach his/her goals. Setting goals for the client may undermine the counseling and his/her motivation to change.
- Ask the patient if he or she feels comfortable involving a support system. If so, bring these individuals into counseling to help "check" and motivate the patient when he or she needs it.
- Stress the importance of keeping an accurate journal, to include information about food, biological markers (including blood glucose measurements, if necessary), and emotions about food and/or goals.

Effective communication

Effective communication is evidenced by mutual understanding, body language, and follow-through on information discussed. Some characteristics of effective communication including the following:

- Good eye-contact. Eye contact shared by both parties conveys interest and understanding between the individuals. Looking down or away from the presenter may indicate that a topic is not well-understood, is an uncomfortable subject, or needs further discussion.
- Effective oral communication. When communicating orally, it is imperative that all parties understand one another. Slow, clear speech greatly improves understanding and comprehension of material discussed. Additionally, hearing devices and/or translators should be used when necessary.
- Open dialogue. Even when presenting nutritional information to another, an open dialogue is important. Questions asked to and from both individuals helps drive critical points and clarify weakly communicated topics.
- Quiet, undisturbed environment. Communication in any counseling setting is most effective in a quiet environment with little distraction.

Friends and family

Friends and family are an integral part of counseling as they are often the most influential forces in a patient's life. Family may be able to encourage and motivate a client to make changes to his/her diet, and in effect, improve the health of the patient. Additionally, family members and friends may be willing to modify their diet in order to follow the nutritional guidelines set forth for the patient. Friends and family are also a great source of accountability for patients. Not only can these individuals help the patient stay on his/her nutritional plan, but these individuals may also assist in dietary journaling/documentation. This is especially important when the patient has dementia or impaired memory.

Employee Management

Hire & Supervise

Staffing

Staffing is the implementation of a plan which is designed to cover all of the human resources needs. In order to properly staff, one must combine resources, including knowledge, skill, and time, to make an organization, its employees, and its processes effective. Staffing includes such tasks as recruiting, interviewing, and selecting employees. Once a potential employee has been selected, staffing includes hiring the individual and providing employee orientation. Then, while on staff, the employee must receive continued training in order to be effective for the organization, and the manager must ensure employee satisfaction, distribution of benefits, and other tactics in order to encourage retention of all employees. In other words, staffing is the total picture, from recruitment to retention of employees.

A job is defined as the combination of tasks assigned to an employee, an individual who is hired to work for an organization. The employee is held accountable for completing the tasks; these tasks comprise the employee's job. A job may be performed by more than one employee. Sometimes the employees work concurrently, sometimes the employees are hired and terminated and/or resign one after another. For example, there may be more than one dietary manager on staff at a facility at any given time. Perhaps these individuals split the duties of the job; more likely, however, the individuals perform the job duties during different shifts or on different wards. In this case, there are two or more employees filling the same job. That is to say, both individuals are dietary managers for facility X. On the other hand, a facility may decide that their needs are met by having only one dietary manager on staff. When that individual resigns, another dietary manager is hired. In this case, there is only one individual (one employee) performing the job of dietary manager at facility Y.

Job analysis

A job analysis is the breakdown of a job into very specific and detailed tasks. The analysis may take the description of duties from a job description and further define those duties by listing the tasks necessary for completion of each duty. The analysis may also list the frequency by which the tasks should be performed, the time of day those tasks are performed, and the skills necessary to complete the tasks. A job analysis does not, however, include personality characteristics, as they are not actually tasks that are carried out. Rather, personality characteristics define the manner in which those tasks are completed. A job analysis may be helpful in creating a rubric for recruiting, screening, and hiring candidates. Additionally, the analysis is often used to determine salary ranges for employees.

Job descriptions

Job descriptions are powerful tools for the hiring and retention of employees. During the hiring process, for example, a properly and accurately crafted job description helps both the recruiter and the potential employee understand the breadth of the job, including the duties and expectations therein. Job descriptions may guide an interview panel's questions to the potential candidate. Furthermore, the description may help a candidate and/or panel determine whether placing the candidate in that position is realistic. Additionally, job descriptions are helpful to employee retention, in that they provide the employee with a guide of the organization's expectations for that individual. Moreover, a job description is a great tool to provide new employees with; doing so will ensure that the individual is made aware of all his/her responsibilities.

A job description is a detailed listing of the tasks that must be fulfilled by an employee. The description also includes information about when and where the employee may work, qualifications for the job, and working conditions. Elements of a job description include:
- Job title
- Department
- Supervisor/Manager
- Responsibilities
- Duties
- Working conditions
- Qualifications for employment
- Employment conditions
- Salary range
- Date of latest revision

FTE

FTE is the acronym for full time equivalent. A full time employee works an average of 40 hours per week. Thus, a full time equivalent (FTE) is an employee or combination of employees that make up the equivalent of a full time employee, or 40 hours per week. So, the number of FTE's does not necessarily match the number of employees. In some cases, there may be a one-to-one match between employees and FTE's. In other instances, the work force of two, three, or even four individuals may equal one FTE. It is important to note that one need not work the standard work week to be considered an FTE. That is to say, any individual or group of individuals working 40 hours per week is considered an FTE. So, one FTE may work eight hours per day, Monday through Friday while another may work ten hours per day, four days of the week. Both are considered FTE's.

Depending upon the make-up of the organization's staff, one may calculate FTE's using a variety of different data. One full time equivalent:

(8 hours/day) x (5 days/week) x (52 days/year) = 2080 hours per year.

Determine number of FTE's for part-time employees. In this case, there are two employees, each working 30 hours per week. To calculate the number of FTE's, divide the total number of hours worked by 2080, the FTE equivalent:

(2 employees) x (30 hours/week) x (52 weeks/year) / (2080 hours/year) = 1.5 FTE

Then, to find the total number of FTE's, add the FTE's for full-time and part-time employees. So that, if a facility employs one individual, full-time and two individuals at thirty hours per week, the number of FTE's would be calculated using the information above, such that:

$$1 \text{ FTE} + 1.5 \text{ FTE's} = 2.5 \text{ FTE's}$$

To determine the number of FTE's for a period of time, take the total number of labor hours for that period and divide that number by the "prorated" FTE. To find the prorated FTE, divide 2080 [the number of hours comprising one full-time equivalent (FTE)] by the portion of the year that is being evaluated.

For the monthly FTE:

(2080 hours/year) / (12 months/year) = 173.33 hours/month

For the quarterly FTE:

(2080 hours/year) / (4 quarters/year) = 520 hours/quarter

For the biannual (6 months) FTE:

(2080 hours/year) / (2 six-months/year) = 1040 hours/six-months

So, if your organization requires 15,000 labor hours every 6 months, the biannual FTE is calculated as follows:

(15,000 hours) / (1040 hours/FTE) = 14.4 FTE

If the organization required the same number of labor hours over the course of a year, the number for FTE's would be calculated as follows:

(15,000 hours) / (2080 hours/FTE) = 7.2 FTE

Exempt and non-exempt employees

There are two types of employees, exempt employees and non-exempt employees. The type of employee determines pay and benefits given to the individuals. Exempt employees are individuals who are on salary and do not receive overtime when working more than a forty hour week. It is expected that the employee will fulfill the requirements of the job, regardless of the number of hours it takes. On the other hand, non-exempt employees do receive overtime pay when working an abnormally long day and/or work-week. State and federal law dictate the conditions of overtime, to include work hours and compensation for working the extra hours.

Staff scheduling

Scheduling a staff is a difficult but important task. Scheduling must first and foremost meet the needs of a facility. A schedule should be developed such that an adequate work force is available to fulfill the labor needs, without over-scheduling employees. The schedule must be cost-effective and labor-effective. The needs and desires of the employees should be secondary to those of the facility. Obviously, the more a manager can cater to employee preference, the greater the employee satisfaction; however, a manager cannot be perpetually concerned with fulfilling employee wishes. Moreover, schedules should be developed in accordance to facility operating procedure and guidelines. Those guidelines may dictate the length of shifts, number of employees scheduled at any given time or for a specific department, make-up of shift employees (number of managers, exempt employees, and non-exempt employees), etc.

Creative scheduling is a skill that is acquired with practice. Such scheduling is done in a manner that most effectively balances labor needs and minimizes labor costs. Creative scheduling may require the implementation of various timed shifts, staggered shifts, split-shifts, and other similar methods. Vary shift times to meet the needs of the facility. Use part-time employees to fill three, four, and five hour shifts, rather than scheduling an individual for eight hours, which may include downtime. Stagger employees such that start times vary by thirty minutes to an hour. If done appropriately, shift staggering will provide the largest labor force during the highest period of need. Split shifts are when shifts are broken by a period of time-off, so that an employee may work four hours in the morning, followed by a few hours off and another four hour shift.

Scheduling conflicts are inevitable. A manager must always work for the benefit of the facility and that means remaining flexible. Illness, employee resignation and/or termination, unexpected leave and vacation, and other scheduling conflicts will arise. In order to mediate scheduling conflicts, it is helpful to have employees who are available on a per diem basis, temporary and on-call employees are also helpful in filling unexpected voids left by other employees. In addition to unexpected conflicts, there will always be other scheduling conflicts resulting from employee preference. When scheduling employees, try to accommodate time-off requests. In the event that multiple time-off requests are received, grant the leave on a first-come, first-served basis. Do not play favorites; be fair to all employees, and keep the needs of the facility as the priority.

Cross-training

Cross-training is a method employed by many organizations to increase the efficiency and proficiency of a staff. When cross-training is properly utilized and implemented, staff members are trained to perform more than one job. Generally, staff members who perform similar jobs are trained on each other's duties and position. When done well, cross-training enables staff to step up in another's absence. Thus, in the event of an unexpected absence, the facility may continue to operate in a manner that is consistent with prior operating procedure and efficiency. In the event of an employee termination, cross-training empowers the facility to do a thorough search for a new employee as the tasks of the unfilled position are still being completed.

Personnel organization chart

A personnel organization chart is a chart that illustrates the personnel structure of an organization. The purpose of the chart is to help employees understand the organization's hierarchy and grouping of employees, which enables individuals with the ability to address questions, concerns, and personnel matters to the correct individuals. Below is an example of a personnel organization chart.

Absences and tardiness

Every manager will run into issues with employee absences and tardiness over the course of their tenure as manager. It is important to deal with these instances as prescribed by the facility's operating procedure, and, in this case, guidance in regards to procedure will most often be found in the human resources department. All absences and tardiness should be documented by the manager and entered into the employee's personnel file. Repeat infractions should also be noted. It is advisable to counsel tardy employees in regards to the organization's procedure and consequences of subsequent absences or tardiness. If an employee's absence or tardiness becomes frequent or surpasses the employee's "allowance," he or she may need to be terminated.

Job routine

A job routine is a timetable, per se, for each work day, and one may be developed for each job position. An example job routine is below:
- 5:00 AM - Report to work in uniform /ready to work, clock in, collect and sort completed menu cards
- 5:30 AM - Prepare tray-line station with utensils, food, etc.
- 6:00 AM - Begin tray-line serving
- 7:00 AM - Assist in tray delivery
- 7:30 AM - Clean kitchen prep area

The job routine would continue to be outlined for the entire work shift. It is important to note that the job routine is the schedule for tasks to be completed within a shift whereas the work schedule outlines the shifts for which an employee is scheduled during a given week/period.

Minimizing overtime

Overtime is always costly to an employer as laws require that employees who work hours beyond that regularly allowed by law be paid one and a half times their normal hourly wage. Therefore, authorizing overtime on a frequent basis may cost the organization more money than if another FTE (full-time equivalent) were added to the staff. Additionally, employees who work excessive hours and shifts are more likely to experience tiredness and fatigue during the shift, which may result in on-the-job errors and inefficiency. To minimize overtime, ensure that your staff is large enough to accommodate all of the organization's needs and try to have on-call employees available to fill in for absent staff. Use job descriptions, analyses, and routines to accurately estimate the task completion time and to properly schedule staff in order to fulfill facility needs. Also, monitor staff through daily interaction as well as performance appraisals to ensure employee efficiency.

Age and marital status

Employment law forbids many questions from being asked by the interviewer to the interviewee. These restrictions are in the best interest of fairness and to minimize discrimination. Questions that cannot lawfully be asked during an interview include the following:
- Information about a name change and/or maiden name
- Birthplace of applicant and/or relatives.
- Requirement to produce a birth certificate, naturalization record, or other similar document
- Applicant's age. *Note: The interviewer may inquire if an interviewee is at least the age necessary for employment. For example, he or she could ask, "Are you at least 16 years of age?"

- Questions regarding the applicant's marital and family status. This includes lines of questioning about a spouse's name, employment status, employer, etc. Additionally, an interviewer may not question an applicant in regards to his/her children or plan to have children.
- Inquiries regarding religion or practices therein

Physical characteristics

In the interest of minimizing discrimination, questions about a person's physical stature and characteristics are off limits during an employment interview. Question topics that are illegal to inquire about during an interview include:
- Race or color of skin
- Height
- Weight
- Sex, including questions about gender, one's ability and/or plan to have children and/or use of or feelings about birth control.
- Requirement that a photograph be submitted with the job application/resume or during/after an interview. An applicant may be given the option to submit a photograph.
- Health questions that do not directly pertain to the individual's ability to perform the job duties. Furthermore, women may not be required to undergo any type of gynecological exam.

United States citizenship

An interviewer may question an applicant in regards to his/her American citizenship, intentions to become a citizen if not already one, as well as his/her legal right to reside and work in the United States. The interviewer may also ask an applicant whether he or she has the ability to fluently write or speak foreign languages. An interviewer cannot, however, ask an applicant general questions about an applicant's citizenship (including date of citizenship and/or country to which he or she is a citizen), country of origin, or citizenship/country of origin of the applicant's relatives. An employer cannot require that an applicant produce naturalization papers.

Experience and education

Interview questions regarding an individual's education and/or work experience are paramount to determining whether an individual is qualified for the position that he or she is applying to. These questions may include inquiries into an individual's academic, professional, and technical training as well as information about previous work or volunteer experience and foreign travel. The interviewer must be careful, however, not to elicit information that would provide a basis for discrimination. For example, asking a potential employee about his/her affiliation to organizations which may indicate the individual's religious preferences, race, ethnicity, or any other personal and identifying information may result in discrimination. Therefore, it is prudent to avoid asking an individual to list all organizations with which he or she has been affiliated. A more appropriate question would be, "Please tell me about your experience, to include work, volunteer, and other experience that has equipped you to perform this job."

Discrimination

Discrimination is the act of treating an individual differently because of his/her race, class, beliefs, sex, or any other category. Even if treatment is favorable, it may still be discrimination. Treatment of all individual's must be based upon that individual's merit, experience, and interactions with others. Managers must be particularly vigilant to prevent workplace discrimination as it is illegal, on all levels—educational, organizational, and governmental—and in all states. It is imperative that managers not tolerate discrimination between peers as well as in supervisor and subordinate relationships. The United States Equal Employment Opportunity Commission enforces law regarding discrimination and has stated that ignorance is not an excuse for discrimination. Therefore, anyone with questions regarding the legality of organizational policy and treatment of employees should reference state and federal employee law resources.

Bona fide occupational qualifications

Bona fide occupational qualifications (BFOQ) are qualifications, which under different circumstances may be considered discriminatory, that are absolutely necessary to perform the functions of a job. Rarely, if ever, would these qualifications apply, and when using BFOQ as a justification against a claim of discrimination, the qualifications must be absolute. For example, defending that only male physical education teachers will be hired on the basis that men are more athletic than women is illegal. However, requiring that each school employ both a male and a female physical education teacher on the basis that students must have same-sex supervision in the locker room is a BFOQ. In this example, there may be a time when the school is only hiring a male teacher or a female teacher.

Legal issues and legislation

Disabilities

According to the American with Disabilities Act (ADA) a disability is defined as "A physical or mental impairment that substantially limits one or more major life activities of such individuals; a record of such an impairment; or being regarded as having such an impairment." The ADA protects individual with a wide range of disabilities from discrimination by regulating that "reasonable accommodation" be made for these individuals so that they may utilize the facility and (in the case of employees) perform their jobs. Accommodations may include structural modifications to allow access to the facility and restrooms, the organization's good and services, as well as any other goods, service, or facility managed by the organization. In the case of an employee, certain job duties may need to be modified to accommodate the employee's disability. All organizations with at least fifteen employees must comply with ADA regulations.

Sexual harassment

Sexual harassment is defined as any conduct or action that is unwelcome and sexual in nature, to include all acts that are physical or verbal. Additionally, sexual harassment may be perceived through the use of various items used to decorate one's workspace (inappropriate and sexual photographs, calendars, slogans, etc.). The United States Equal Employment Opportunity Commission guidelines suggest that in the event that sexual harassment occurs, the harassment should be reported to a supervisor, investigated, and the legality of such acts should be determined. The accused individual should be confronted and given the opportunity to defend him/herself. At that time, and after seeking legal counsel, the organization should determine what, if any, disciplinary action will be taken. Managers should always consult the organization's policy and human resources department before taking any action on a sexual harassment claim. Furthermore employees should be provided information and educated about the organization's sexual harassment policy. Clearly defining acts that constitute sexual harassment will serve to minimize, if not altogether eliminate, the occurrence of such acts.

Fair Labor Standards Act

The Fair Labor Standards Act (FLSA) establishes minimum wage (to include a "tip credit" for employees who receive tips), a forty hour week, overtime pay (1.5 times regular wages) for non-exempt employees, employment/wage record keeping policies, and child-labor laws. Child labor laws include restrictions on minimum age of an employee, number of hours a child laborer may work (dependent upon school session), and hours of the day in which children may be assigned shifts. The FLSA regulations apply to all laborers in the United States of America. Individual states may have regulations in addition to those put forth by the Fair Labor Standards Act.

Workers compensation

Workers Compensation is a component of the Federal Employment Compensation Act, though it is administered by state statutes. The purpose of workers compensation is to limit an employer's liability in the event that an employee is either injured or killed on the job. Provisions may include compensation for medical bills and lost income. In the event of an employee's death, workers compensation may award benefits to the surviving spouse and/or next of kin. In the event of an employee injury, follow the protocol established by the state's legislation. This information should be readily available through the state's Department of Labor.

Family and Medical Leave Act

The Family and Medical Leave Act (FMLA) is federal legislation which protects an eligible employee's job for up to twelve weeks in any twelve month period. The purposes for which this time off may be granted and protected include the following:
- Birth and care of a newborn child
- Placement of a foster child or adopted son or daughter
- Care of an immediate family member who is suffering from a serious health condition
- Leave requested to cope with and/or recover from a serious medical condition, which prevents an individual from performing his/her work duties

*Note: The Family and Medical Leave Act does not guarantee paid time off, only unpaid time off. Questions regarding the Family and Medical Leave Act should be directed to the Department of Labor.

Federal Unemployment Tax Act

The Federal Unemployment Tax Act (FUTA) works in conjunction with state unemployment policies to provide income to individuals who are unemployed and are not at fault for losing their jobs. For example, an individual who voluntarily resigns from a job and/or is terminated due to disciplinary action does not qualify to receive unemployment benefits. On the other hand, an individual who is laid off due to budget cuts would qualify for the benefit. Those qualifying for unemployment assistance must actively be seeking future employment. Unemployment taxes are collected by federal and state governments and in addition to providing income for unemployed individuals are used to provide services to individuals seeking employment assistance. Unemployment taxes may be levied on the employer and/or the employee, depending upon state regulations.

<u>Equal pay</u>
Several legislative acts, including the Equal Pay Act, The Civil Rights Act, Age Discrimination in Employment Act, and Americans with Disabilities Act, mandate equal pay for employees performing jobs requiring "equal skill, effort, and responsibility." Differences in employee compensation are only allowed when based solely on job performance, to include employee seniority, merit, and quality of work. Additionally, employees who complete a greater quantity of work in the same time as other employees may be rewarded with greater compensation. Any type of pay discrimination based upon sex, religion, race, and other characteristics outside of job performance are illegal.

Performance standards

Performance standards are benchmarks which describe the desired work output and outcomes achieved by an employee. These standards should be realistic and quantifiable, such that the employee has a reasonable goal for which he or she can strive on a daily basis. Performance standards are typically developed by defining the standard and the rubric by which the standard is judged. The rubric must be designed such that it provides a clear, objective measurement of each standard. Performance standards should be developed for each task listed within an employee's job description. Once the employee is provided the standard operating procedures and has been trained, it is then reasonable to evaluate the employee's performance based upon the rubric for each performance standard.

Standard operating procedure

Standard operating procedure, also referred to as SOPs, is the facility's prescribed method to address and complete each task, position, and facility procedure. SOPs must be made available to all employees, so that every individual may easily reference the procedure. SOPs are essential to organizations in that they promote uniform policy by which employees may address tasks, questions, concerns, and procedures. Additionally SOPs are integral to defining and measuring performance standards, which in turn are essential to performance evaluations. SOPs should frequently be revisited so that all procedures may be updated to promote the utmost accuracy and efficiency for the entire organization. When updated, employees should be educated as to the changes to the procedure and new SOPs should be posted accordingly.

Motivation

Motivation is any influence which drives an individual to complete a task or to work towards a goal. Individuals may be motivated by a variety of incentives and in a vast array of manners. An effective manager will learn how to motive his/her employees such that they are eager and willing to perform the tasks of their jobs and take pride in that performance. It is imperative that the expectations placed on an employee are realistic and laced with reasonable goals. If not, the employee will not know the joy and satisfaction that results from a job well-done, and motivation will be severely lacking. Managers may adopt a variety of policies, to include efforts as elaborate as financial and time-off reward incentives and as simple as personal expressions of appreciation and employee recognition.

McClelland and his fellow researchers identified three primary human needs. According to their research, those needs include the need for power, for affiliation, and for achievement. It is proposed that each person is motivated more strongly by one of those needs than the others, such that you may have one employee who is empowered by increased perception of his/her power, one who is motivated by his/her affiliation with the organization and other employees, and another who is motivated by achievement—setting and meeting various goals. Managers striving to motivate employees may try to discern which of the three "needs" is primary to each individual. Once the need has identified, it may be effective for managers to assign tasks in a manner which allows the employee the opportunity to fulfill his/her need—power, affiliation, or achievement.

Vroom's theory postulates that an individual is motivated by a careful evaluation of the effort necessary to put forth a successful performance which will then lead to a positive outcome. So, by Vroom's account, employees are motivated by outcomes which will elicit positive consequences, such as time-off, increased pay, employee recognition, etc. In keeping with his theory, managers can motivate employees by assigning tasks requiring a realistic and reasonable amount of effort. Furthermore, employees must be assured that they will be rewarded for a job well-done. Even tasks requiring extra hours and effort from an employee may be greeted with a high level of excitement and willingness if the employees know that the effort will bear fruit.

The equity theory is one in which an individual's performance may be largely enhanced or disrupted by his/her perception of how other colleagues are treated in comparison to him/herself. So, if an employee perceives that he is being treated as well or better than other employees, he or she will continue to work hard and will likely maintain if not strengthen his/her work ethic. On the other hand, if an employee feels like he or she does not receive recognition for his/her efforts, or if the recognition pails in comparison to the recognition others receive, the employee may fail to perform. In fact, if an individual feels as though he or she is being treated unfairly, it is likely that the individual may become disruptive to the organization as a whole.

Work climate

Work climate is the term used to describe the general well-being and over-arching emotion that runs through a work environment. In other words, work climate is the environment which shapes employee morale. A positive work climate is one in which all employees are given respect, feel valued, and work as a team. A positive work environment will, by nature, be one that is encouraging and motivating to the employees. The climate is welcoming to new employees and is free from constant competition. Conversely, a negative work climate is generally one riddled with dissatisfied employees, poor work ethic, and disrespect. This type of climate breeds low morale and may result in decreased productivity, poor customer service, and high employee turnover.

Team building

Team building is an important contributor to positive morale. When employees feel as if they are a member of the team, they are likely to take greater pride in their work and share their accomplishments. Furthermore, team building aids in keeping any one employee from feeling overwhelmed and under appreciated. Moreover, working as a team promotes respect within the organization (both peer-to-peer as well as a respect for the organizational hierarchy). To promote the staff as a team, celebrate group accomplishments and highlight the bigger picture rather than just individual achievement. Include all staff in relevant meetings and try to host an annual retreat for the staff to engage in team-building opportunities. As a manager, one must be available to his/her entire team so that all employees feel comfortable bringing questions, concerns, and suggestions to the management's attention. Moreover, a manager should help mediate employee conflict as well as compliment impressive teamwork.

Effective feedback

Feedback is essential to employee performance and staff morale. Feedback is the act of communicating both positive and negative criticisms, advice, and compliments to members of your staff. All feedback should be handled delicately. Giving members of your team effective feedback is a skill that is achieved with practice. Feedback should be delivered to correct a problem as well as to compliment an employee on a job well-done. Feedback is best received when given immediately and in private (especially when giving negative feedback). It is important that feedback focus on the action or the person's behavior, and the concern should be specific. A manager should avoid laying blame on the employee and should allow the employee to respond to the manager's concern/compliment. Additionally, it is important to direct, or, in some cases redirect, an employee to the appropriate actions giving clear and precise instruction. If necessary, demonstrate or pair the employee with another staff member to demonstrate the proper procedure. Moreover, a manager should make him/herself available for employee questions. Finally, after delivering feedback, it is advisable to provide the employee with positive feedback when he or she improves (or continues excellent) performance.

Performance review

A performance review is the evaluation of an employee and his/her job proficiency. This is an opportunity for a manager to meet with his/her employees to provide structured feedback. Performance reviews are essential to setting goals, promoting employee growth, and ensuring that employees have the education and tools necessary to perform their jobs. Additionally, performance reviews provide data for employees' personal files, a basis for wage structure and increases, and documentation supporting promotion and/or termination. It is important, however, that continuous feedback be provided to employees so that they are not blind-sighted by negative feedback during a performance review. Doing so is unfair to the employee as the review will be entered into his/her personnel file.

The frequency with which performance reviews are carried out varies based upon organizational needs and policy. Performance reviews may be carried out as frequently as the organization deems necessary. Many organizations consider the first sixty to ninety days of a new-hire's employment a probationary period. Generally, a performance review is carried out at the end of the probationary period and is often followed by a review after six-months, around the employee's one-year anniversary, and annually thereafter. It is advisable that management review employee performance at least once a year. Allowing too much time to pass between reviews may hinder employee morale as staff members may feel ignored and unnoticed.

An open-ended performance review is one in which the manager may write out an employee's strengths and weaknesses without a specific guide for evaluation. The manager

- 44 -

may also include notes regarding suggestions for improvement or benchmarks that should be met in order to be considered for promotion. On the other hand, an objective based performance review is one in which the manager and employee have mutually determined objectives, or goals, to be met during the review period by the employee. The employee is then evaluated on his or her ability to complete the objectives and the proficiency with which he or she met the stated goals. At the end of the evaluation, the employee and manager again set certain objectives for which the employee will be responsible during the next reporting period.

There are many different performance review formats, and the facility should choose a format that appropriately serves the needs of an organization. Some of the pros and cons of a checklist performance review format are listed below:

Pros:

- Lists specific areas of evaluation rated on a scale; ensures employees are evaluated using the same qualifying characteristics
- Generally offers room for specific comments
- May be quickly filled out by managers
- Easy to see employee shortcomings

Cons:

- Because of easy format, managers may not be as thoughtful as they should be when evaluating an employee
- May fail to elicit particular strengths of an individual, including his/her ability to perform certain job tasks
- Various managers may weight scale differently, leading to discrepancy

A forced-choice performance review is a general evaluation that lists employee qualities and presents a rubric on which the individual may be graded. Each grade of the rubric is specifically defined so that terms like "superior" and "poor" are less ambiguous to the individual performing the evaluation. Some pros and cons of a forced-choice performance review are listed below:

Pros:

- Employees are evaluated on the same qualifiers
- Rubric scale allows for greater consistency, especially when more than one person is evaluating employees
- Format is less time-consuming than an open-ended review

Cons:

- Manager is less likely to add additional modifiers to the rubric and may not be as thoughtful as when using an open-ended format
- May fail to elicit employee's individual strengths, both in character and job performance
- Manager may be less likely to add additional comments to the review and/or take time to set goals with the employee

An open-ended performance review is an evaluation in which the supervisor writes in his/her comments regarding an employee's performance. Unlike other formats, this type of review is not generally scale or rubric based. Some pros and cons of this type of performance review format are listed below:

Pros:
- Gives manager the opportunity to pinpoint and elaborate upon employee's strengths and weaknesses
- May facilitate a comprehensive discussion regarding employee's performance, goal-setting, promotion, etc.
- Format is often designed to direct managers so that a well-rounded assessment is performed

Cons:
- Not an effective format if employees are evaluated by more than one individual as it is too objective
- Managers may fail to comment on important aspects of employees performance
- If a manager's use of language is ambiguous, the review may be difficult to understand and/or misinterpreted

Because performance reviews should be entered into employees' permanent personnel files, it is important to give every employee the opportunity to formally review and comment on the evaluation. In some cases, an employee may enter information regarding future goals and objectives. Other times, employees may choose to include a rebuttal of or justification for negative evaluations, which may or may not include information about training (or a lack thereof) and how that individual perceives his/her treatment by management and/or other employees. At the very least, employees should sign off on performance reviews in order to acknowledge that the information therein was reviewed by both the manager and employee.

Corrective action

Corrective action is the process that is carried out by a manager to modify an employee's performance and/or change his/her behavior. It is important to note that corrective action does not exclusively apply to negative situations. Every facility should have a policy for carrying out corrective action. Generally, corrective action will be documented and entered into the employee's personnel file. Corrective action should focus on the behavior or performance, not the individual. Moreover, it is advisable for the manager to help the employee develop a plan to avoid future problems relating to the corrective action. As with performance reviews, both employees and manager should sign the corrective action documentation to acknowledge that the information was received (even if the employee does not agree with the action).

Progressive discipline

Progressive discipline is a series of steps taken to modify employee performance or behavior. Depending on the standard operational procedure of a facility, the number of steps and extent of progressive discipline widely varies. Generally, progressive discipline begins with notation of corrective action. When an employee fails to improve performance, additional corrective action may be taken. Failed performance/behavioral improvement may result penalties including a wage deduction, suspension, and termination. It is imperative that all corrective action be documented and acknowledged by both manager and employee. In the event of employee termination, documentation of corrective action may be necessary to justify the termination.

Employee assistance programs

Many institutions have some sort of organized employee assistance program. These programs are designed to assist employees, and in some cases, their families, when dealing with a variety of issues, to include drug and alcohol addictions, domestic violence, harassment, and other personal and family issues. Depending upon the type of organization, the employee assistance program may be administered by the organization or contracted to an outside organization/provider. Employee assistance programs are beneficial to organizations in that provide employees with the psychological assistance they need to be productive in their personal, social, and professional lives. Moreover, such programs are likely to breed greater loyalty among employees.

Employee recognition

Employee recognition is essential to promoting and maintaining high morale at any business. There are various means by which a manager can recognize his/her employees, some of those means are listed below:
- Verbally provide positive feedback and expressions of appreciation
- Ask employees to nominate peers for various awards and recognition
- Make comment cards available for customers to recognize employees
- Acknowledge employees for outstanding service, attendance, and years of service to an organization
- Honor employees with time off, certificates of appreciate, plaques, receptions, luncheons, and parties
- Surprise employees with small, appropriate gifts and comments from those they have served
- Allow employees to bring a child with them to work once a year

Employee termination

Termination of an employee is a delicate matter and should be handled with respect and grace. Generally, termination of an employee should be preceded by documented corrective action. However, there are times when immediate employee termination is warranted, such as when an employee blatantly ignores the rules of the facility, endangers fellow employees or customers, or commits an illegal act. Other circumstances warranting employee termination include chronic absenteeism or tardiness, insubordination, fraudulently documenting time on the job, misuse of the facility's property or resources, an employee's unwillingness to perform functions of the job, and his/her inability to modify behavior addressed by corrective action/progressive discipline. In all cases documentation of violations to the organization's policy as well as any corrective action and/or counseling that has occurred is essential.

Develop Personnel & Communication

Illness of food service employees

The following symptoms should be reported by food service employees to his/her manager prior to working his/her shift:
- Sore throat with fever
- Diarrhea
- Vomiting
- Jaundice
- Open wound, lesion, or boil that is oozing or seeping pus

Open wounds and lesions may not present a risk of transmittable foodborne illness if an impermeable barrier (such as a glove) protects the area from coming into contact with food, utensils, and serving equipment. After an employee reports his/her symptoms, it is then the manager's responsibility to determine whether the employee poses a risk to transmit a foodborne illness and if that employee should be restricted or excluded from food service until his/her symptoms clear.

The following illness diagnoses and/or recent history of exposure to the following should be reported by food service employees to his/her manager prior to working his/her shift:
- Norovirus
- Hepatitis A virus
- Shigella
- Enterohemorrhagic Escherichia coli (E Coli)
- Shiga toxin-producing Escherichia coli (E Coli)
- Salmonella Thyphi

It is then the responsibility of the manager to notify the health department (or other regulating agency) of the food employee's illness.
*Note: A manager should also notify the health department in the event that an employee reports jaundice.

Hygiene

Proper hand-washing
The FDA Food Code clearly describes the proper hand-washing procedure. The code states that the hands and exposed portions of the arms, to include any prosthetics, must be thoroughly washed for at least twenty seconds, using an approved cleaning solution and at an approved hand-washing sink. The procedure to be followed when washing hands is as follows:
1. Rinse with clean, warm, running water
2. Apply cleaning solution
3. Rub vigorously (creating friction) for 10-15 seconds, paying particular attention to the fingernails and other hard to reach surfaces
4. Rinse with clean, warm, running water
5. Thoroughly dry with paper towel

According to the FDA Food Code, food service employees must wash their hands after each incidence in which they:

- Touch any bare human body part other than the cleaned hands and exposed portion of the arm
- Use the restroom
- Care for or handle service or aquatic animals
- Cough, sneeze, and use a tissue
- Use tobacco, eat, or drink
- Handle soiled utensils, service ware, and kitchen equipment
- Prepare food which may cause cross contamination
- Handle raw food and before handling ready to eat food
- Engage in any other activity that may contaminate their hands

*Note: Food service employees must also wash their hands before putting on gloves.

Food service employees are only to wash their hands in a hand-washing sink. This area should be designated (and clearly marked) for hand-washing, and hand-washing only. An employee should not wash his/her hands in any sink used for cleaning kitchen equipment, utensils, or service ware. Moreover, sinks used for food preparation or cleaning are off limits to hand-washing. The use of a hand-washing sink is mandated by the FDA Food Code, and as such, is scrutinized by regulating agencies.

*Note: Approved antiseptic hand sanitizers/dips/solutions may also be utilized between washes, but these solutions may only be applied after following correct hand-washing procedure at a designated hand-washing sink.

Grooming and accessory regulations

The FDA Food Code regulates personal grooming and accessories of food services employees. According to the code, food service employees are required to have well-groomed fingernails that are trimmed and filed such that the nails are easily cleaned and do not have any rough edges. Furthermore, unless an employee wears gloves, he or she is not allowed to wear fingernail polish or artificial nails while working in food services. The food code also states that food service employees who are doing any sort of food preparation are not allowed to wear jewelry on their hands and arms, with the exception of "a plain ring such as a wedding band." This prohibition also applies to medical-identification jewelry. Additionally, the food code mandates that all outer clothing be clean so as to prevent contamination of the food.

The FDA Food Code requires that all employees who are at risk of contaminating prepared food, utensils, service ware, and food preparation equipment properly cover and restrain all body hair. This policy does not apply to those who pose a minimal risk of food contamination, such as host/hostess, wait staff, counter attendants, and other similar employees. Hair should be pulled back away from the employee's face and covered with a hat, hair net, or other similar device. Additionally, employees with facial hair should appropriately restrain hair using a beard restraint or hair net. For this reason, many facilities adopt policies requiring employees to be clean shaven, except when doing so interferes with one's religious beliefs. Moreover, employees should minimize exposure to body hair by wearing covering clothing. The FDA Food Code also states that employees who "experience persistent sneezing, coughing, or a runny nose that causes discharge from the eyes, nose, or mouth" may not work with food, service ware, utensils, or preparation equipment.

<u>Consuming beverages in kitchen/food preparation area</u>
A food service employee may consume beverages while in the food preparation area if and only if the employee complies with the FDA Food Code. Beverages must be consumed from a closed container that is properly handled to prevent contamination of the employee's hand, the container itself, and any food preparation equipment, utensils, service ware, or the food itself.
*Note: At no time should a food service employee consume food or use tobacco products while on duty.

Change

Change is essential to the life and growth of any organization. Sometimes change may be as simple as making small revisions to the daily routine or it may be as large as an organizational reorganization. Regardless of the measure of change, many employees may be resistant to make changes. Resistance to change is a natural reaction and as such should be addressed by managers. Some of the many reasons that employees may resist change include:
- Fear or anxiety about changes to come and their ability to meet new expectations
- Bruised egos; some employees may feel that the desire to change is a reflection upon their previous performances
- Anxiety about relationship dynamics, especially if employees will be working with new individuals
- Questions about their new place within the organization and job stability
- Dissatisfaction with inconveniences brought about by the changes
- Lack of confidence in managers and their plans to restructure the department/organization
- Loss of independence

A manager can adopt a variety of methods to help guide his/her employees through organizational change. Some basic tactics that should be employed include:
- Discuss with employees the reasons for change. If employees understand why change is necessary for the growth of their organization, they may be more willing to partake in the changes.
- Use internal marketing to sell the change to employees; make it an exciting opportunity
- Consider employee fears and anxieties and address these in the context of change
- Allow employees the opportunity to share concerns, feelings, etc.
- Tell employees what is expected of them during and after the change; describe how the organization will support them (i.e., additional training, accommodations, etc.)
- Ask employees to assist in change process and provide feedback regarding change; likewise, be available to answer questions and address concerns throughout the process

Organizations should be continuously evolving, and therefore, change in inherent. While small changes may happen daily and without a catalyst, larger departmental or organizational changes must be well-thought out and developed before being implemented. Change may be necessary when an organization encounters any of the following issues:
- Lack of morale, respect, or motivation among employees and managers
- Organization is no longer cost effective
- Products/menus and attitudes becoming repetitive, lackadaisical, and stale

- Organization lacks diversity, whether in employee dynamics or product output
- Processes and employees fail to meet expectations of organization
- Consensus among employees and/or management that change is necessary

Conflict

Conflict is an inevitable aspect of every working relationship. Conflicts may range from being very minor and having little to no effect on working relationships to being extremely disruptive to the entire organization. Most conflict can be mediated such that both parties come to an agreement or understanding. However, there are certain issues that are directly tied to a person's beliefs and feelings that cannot be mediated. These issues may be discussed, and even debated, but are not generally negotiable:

- Personal beliefs, including those relating to religion, sexual preference, cultural observances, etc.
- Feelings or perceptions, including those of anger, hurt, blame, low self-confidence/self-esteem
- Confidence and trust in fellow employees, managers, and the organization as a whole
- Personal values, morals, and spiritual decisions

It is a manager's responsibility to help mediate employee conflict, and he or she should follow the organization's (human resources) procedure to assist employees in this manner. Generally speaking, a manager can mediate employee conflict if he or she has respect for all parties involved and remains unbiased. When mediating employee conflict, a manager should invite all parties to participate in the mediation, to include being present and being given the opportunity to speak during each session. During mediation, a manager should give the conflicted parties the opportunity to come to a mutually agreeable solution, including a resolution process to which all parties will commit. It may take several mediation sessions for the parties to come to an agreement. In the event that the parties are unable to agree to a solution, the manager may need to step out of the role of mediator and implement what he or she believes to be a fair solution, taking into account all of the perspectives discussed during mediation.

Authoritative management style

An authoritative management style is one in which the manager acts with full authority. He or she makes decisions in what he or she believes is the best interest of the organization and his/her employees. Authoritative managers may seek the input of employees but do not let the employees opinions dictate the decisions that they make. While authoritative managers can appear very powerful, this management style can be detrimental to an organization as it excludes employees. Such exclusion of employee may detrimentally affect employee morale. Additionally, an authoritative management style impedes communication between employees and management, which can adversely affect the manager's knowledge regarding employee wellbeing and satisfaction. Furthermore, employees may fail to perform for an authoritative manager if they do not agree with his/her decisions.

Participative management style

A participative management style is one characterized by a high level of interaction between the manager and his/her subordinates. A participative manager is more likely to get his/her hands dirty and work alongside the organization's personnel. This type of relationship empowers the manager as he or she is more directly involved in employee communication and more readily relates to employee conflict, disputes, and dissatisfaction. Additionally, the manager is able to set an example through his/her actions for other employees to follow. While a participative style is likely to create greater morale among employees than an authoritative style, a manager who employs this method of management risks losing control of his/her employees.

Proactive and reactive management styles

If one is proactive, he or she anticipates future development, cause-and-effect relationships, and other predicted outcomes. Thus, a proactive manager anticipates problems and the need for change. As a proactive individual, this manager will actively work to circumvent problems before they arrive. Such anticipatory action is encouraging to employees as the manager actively works to avoid conflict and problems in the workplace. On the other hand, a person who is reactive is one who responds to a stimulus or situation that has already played out. Conversely, a reactive manager makes decisions based upon past. This type of management style is completely ineffective and puts undue stress on employees and the organization as a whole.

Meetings

Meetings are important to the organization of any group. Meetings allow for the passing of information, the discussion of ideas, and meetings provide time for group brainstorms. Additionally, meetings are the perfect forum for sharing organizational goals, policy, and changes with employees as well as addressing fears and questions relating to those topics. That being said, meetings can be very expensive for an organization as well as for individuals who are attending from outside organizations, as everyone is being paid for their time spent in the meeting. Additionally, transportation costs for those traveling to the meeting location must be factored in. Therefore, meetings should be carefully planned and scheduled to minimize the time and maximize the benefit to the organization.

There are a variety of reasons that a manager may choose to hold meetings. Meetings may be used as an opportunity to build and strengthen a team. Thus, at meetings, team members may share skills, ideas, and project milestones. Furthermore, the team may take part in team-building activities, which highlight individual's strengths. Meetings may also be used to introduce and convey changes to policies and procedures or to orient new employees. Additionally, a manager may choose to hold a meeting in order to train employees or continue employee education. Meetings may also be used as a tool for manager's to "take the pulse" of the organization and employees' morale. Whatever the reason for calling a meeting, it is important that all meetings have set agendas and objectives such that they are a productive part of everyone's professional experience.

According to the Dietary Manager's Association and study guide author, Susan Davis Allen, there are six steps to planning a departmental meeting. Those steps are as follows:

1. Prepare a preliminary agenda
2. Announce meeting to those invited to attend. Be sure to give all staff members ample notice. It is also helpful to send attendees a reminder just before the meeting.
3. Work with other managers and presenters to further develop the meeting agenda
4. Hold the meeting
5. Prepare and disseminate meeting minutes to all relevant staff
6. Develop a plan of action to meet the needs and goals discussed during the meeting

Meetings serve a variety of purposes; therefore, the meeting's agenda should dictate who is invited (or required) to attend each meeting. When planning a meeting, the organizer should consider the goals of the session and then all relevant personnel should be invited to attend. For example, if a manager would like to convey information, such as changes to employee benefits, he or she should invite all personnel in the organization (or his department) to attend. On the other hand, if a manager would like to brainstorm ways in which the tray-line process could be more efficient, it would be more appropriate to include only tray-line employees and supervisors. A meeting organizer should resist the urge to include everyone, just for the sake of contribution. Because the organization must pay all employees their respective wages regardless of how time is spent, meetings can be very expensive to an organization, especially when unnecessary personnel are in attendance. Additionally, too many unnecessary voices may lead to meeting chaos.

Meeting documentation, or meeting minutes, are an important aspect of meeting organization. Meeting minutes are an official record of the information passed and discussed during the meeting. These documents serve as a means of communicating policies and changes to members of the organization, and they serve as a reminder of all action items. Thus, meeting documentation should include the following information:

- Meeting title/name
- Meeting date, time (start and ending), and location
- Meeting attendees, with notation acknowledging meeting leader/organizer, recorder, guests, and other important participants
- Discussion notes; these should be written such that key points are obvious and extraneous notes are brief
- Action items with party responsible for completing each task noted
- Deadlines for action items
- Time, date, and location of follow-up meeting (if applicable)

An agenda is a simple outline and pseudo-schedule for a meeting. Thus, the agenda should list the topics to be discussed, in the order that they are to be discussed. Often, managers will also include specific subtopics on the agenda to help focus a discussion. Agendas are an effective time management tool in that they direct the meeting and help individuals stay on task. It is important that the meeting organizer determine the amount of time necessary to cover each agenda item and convey this to those present. Again, this helps a meeting stay productive and on-course.

If possible, it is beneficial for the meeting organizer to inform the invited meeting attendees in regards to the agenda items in advance. Doing so allows participants the opportunity to do research, brainstorm, and prepare their thoughts prior to the discussion.

Effective meetings depend upon the effective communication of those present. This communication relies upon participation of all meeting attendees and respect for one another's opinions. Ensure all meeting participants have the opportunity to contribute their ideas by directly asking people for their opinions. If there is an individual who is particularly talkative, acknowledge his/her ideas, and ask other team members if they would like to contribute. In the event that the group is stuck on a particular topic, consider "tabling it," or leaving the topic open for the next meeting, so that individuals can more thoroughly examine the issue. Additionally, one may direct the group to come to a consensus through use of a reminder that only a certain amount of time has been allocated for the topic. In the event that the group gets off-course during a meeting, bring the group back to the topic by reiterating the objectives of the meeting.

Effective presentations

Effective and entertaining presentation of material can make the difference between true understanding of the information conveyed and a sleepy audience. Below are some tips to developing and delivering an effective presentation:

- Use graphics, audio-visual equipment, and other props to augment the presentation only
- A presenter should speak loudly and clearly, carefully enunciating words
- Work the room using eyes and body language; never face away from the audience
- Practice the presentation in advance; be careful to note when props/augments will be used as well as how and when to vary voice tone and pace of speech
- Develop the presentation to meet time constraints; build in time for the audience to ask questions
- Prepare handouts for the audience to help with future recall of the information; avoid, however, passing information before or during the presentation as it may become a distraction

There are many methods that can be employed when presenting information to an audience. Some of those methods and their pros and cons are listed below:

- Lecture: Allows presenter full control of information conveyed but may loose attention of audience as it lacks participation
- Demonstration: Gives audience the opportunity to watch presenter perform a task but lacks hands-on experience for audience members
- Participative presentation: Audience members are asked to participate in the presentation; presenter may loose control of audience and presentation
- Discussion: Invites audience to participate in a discussion; again, presenter may loose control of the audience
- Panel presentation: Several presenters join forces to present and discuss information, often opening to audience for questions. This type of presentation can be problematic if the panel has not adequately coordinated and prepared.
- Case studies: Specific details of an example situation are presented to the audience for discussion. Treatment opinions may differ, and it may be difficult for presenter to effectively recommend course of action.

Organizational communication

Due to the extensive size and network within every organization, there will be a plethora of positive and negative communication occurring. Positive communication is characterized by respectful, accurate, and morale-boosting transfer of information that correctly follows the chain of command, so that information is traveling upwards and downwards through the proper individual. Additionally, the information that is being passed remains the same throughout the levels of communication. Upward communication is the transfer of information from subordinate employees to supervisors. This type of communication is meant to keep management in the loop as well as to file complaints, investigate opportunities, etc. On the other hand, downward communication is when information travels from supervisors to subordinates, again, in an effort to inform. Grapevine communication is when unofficial and/or opinionated information is passed to employees. This type of communication may be initiated and past from peer-to-peer, from subordinate-to-supervisor, and vice versa. It is best to keep employees informed and make management available for questions to avoid grapevine communication.

Effective communication is essential to the well-being of a workplace and the positive morale of an organization's staff. Effective communication is communication that is without gossip and does not depend upon the grapevine for the passing and sharing of information. Rather, effective workplace communication is characterized by open channels that enable both upward and downward communication, such that an employee feels comfortable approaching a supervisor with questions and concerns and a supervisor keeps his/her subordinates informed about organizational policy and changes, whether by meeting or memo. Additionally, effective communication follows the organizational chart, so that an employee reports to his/her direct-line supervisor. If that supervisor is unavailable and/or the employee has an unresolved issue that has previously been addressed with the direct-line supervisor, then that individual should consult his/her supervisor's direct-line supervisor for assistance.

Policy and procedure

A policy is a plan carefully crafted to direct an organization in specific situations and under specific circumstances. Often, policies adopt various procedures to accomplish an overall goal, whether that be to ensure employee satisfaction, organize an efficient tray-line, or reporting a work-related incident. Procedures are the steps or tasks that must be carried out in order to adhere to a policy and/or achieve an end goal. Many organizations craft "policy and procedure" documents which outline or state a specific policy and then list the detailed procedures that are necessary to conform to the policy. It is advisable to create a database and/or binders of policies and procedures that are easily accessed by all employees. Doing so will allow employees to reference the material when necessary.

Policy and procedure documents are essential reference materials for all employees. In order to ensure that employees uniformly perform job tasks, policy and procedure documents must be written. Policy and procedure documents should include the following information:
- A name and/or identifier that is easily recognizable to staff; this may include department name and/or numbers
- Uniform structure so that employees can easily reference and find information in a document

- Revision date; it is important that these documents be periodically revised to ensure efficiency
- Reference information (including information from/about regulatory agencies)
- Statement of policy
- Outline of procedure

Employee orientation

Employee orientation is an essential element to employee training. Orientation is an employee's introduction to his/her job, the tasks it requires, policy and procedures, other employees, and other elements of daily performance. During employee orientation, the new employee should be introduced to fellow colleagues; given the mission statement and objectives of the organization as well as his/her specific job; instructed in regards to working hours, uniform, policies, and procedures; given a tour of the facility as well as the facilities offered to employees; provided with the organizational chart, including information in regards to his/her specific line of authority; and educated in regards to any regulations by which the organization must comply.

Employee orientation and training are essential to an organization as both processes promote employee retention, uniformity among employees, and standards of conduct. Training and orientation also help ensure that employees comply with local, state, and federal regulations and adhere to all policies and procedures set forth by an organization. Additionally, proper training helps prevent employee injuries, misconduct, and harassment.

Some topics that a dietary manager may incorporate in training include the following:
- OSHA Standards
- HIPAA Regulations
- FDA Food Code
- Disaster Preparedness
- Reporting Accidents and/or injury
- Employee Rights
- Harassment definition and policy

Training

Training is only effective if it produces results. Managers can measure the success of training sessions by observing employees to see if procedures and methods covered by the training are being employed. If a manager notices that procedures covered during training are not being utilized, he or she may model the behavior for the employee(s) and/or ask if the staff have any additional questions in regards to the techniques taught. It is important that a manager examine whether information passed in training was actually transferred to and received by the learner. The best training methods are those that allow an individual to participate in the learning. A poor trainer may fail to keep the interest of the staff and/or impart knowledge to individuals. On the other hand, some employees may be altogether uninterested regardless of who attempts to pass the information.

Pre- and post-tests are used to focus an audience and measure the learning that occurred during training. Pre-tests will, for example, highlight the areas in which an employee may be lacking essential knowledge. Thus, when these topics are covered during the training he or she may be more interested and willing to receive the information being presented. Post-test, on the other hand, help measure the amount of learning that took place during the training; this is especially true when a pre-test and post-test are compared. Again, the post-test may act as a catalyst for trainees to ask questions about topics that they did not fully understand. Evaluation forms are great tools to help trainees communicate to management whether training was interesting, effective, and beneficial. It is best to allow trainees the opportunity to write in comments as these may help shape future training sessions. On-the-job training is a form of learning that occurs in the workplace, vice learning from a demonstration or lecture in a classroom/conference room. On-the-job training allows trainees the opportunity to practice and refine skills while on the job and working with real clients. Effective on-the-job training pairs a new hire or trainee with an employee who acts as a mentor. On-the-job is best utilized when the mentor tells the trainee about each aspect of the job and then demonstrates the proper procedure used to address that particular situation/policy. Then, the trainee is given the opportunity to perform the task while being observed. This is the perfect time for the mentor to open the floor for questions and/or positively coach the new hire. On-the-job training will follow this cycle allowing the new employee the opportunity to watch, practice, receive constructive criticism, ask questions, and repeat.

Physical design of a kitchen or workspace

Many factors may influence the design of a food service workspace. Some of those factors include:
- Space
- Budget
- Safety (when working in the work space, accommodating multiple employees, accessibility, etc)
- Local/state/federal codes for kitchen and/or construction
- Menu items/types of foods being prepared and served
- Types of appliances and systems being used by the kitchen
- Energy costs
- Noise, lighting, and temperature control
- Sanitation/Cleanliness
- Proximity to receiving and storage areas
- Number of clients being served at a given time

Ergonomics is the use of scientific knowledge about the human body to create spaces, products, and environments that are comfortable, safe, and healthy for people to use. Because people spend such a large amount of time at work, it is important that all workspaces use ergonomics to increase function, efficiency, health, and comfort for all of their employees. Some ergonomic factors of the workplace include the following:
- Properly built and positioned workstations
- Chairs that promote good posture
- Computer positioning and accessories to increase comfort and natural body positioning
- Adaptive equipment that allows for greater ease of use, handling, and/or decreased repetitive motion
- Accessibility of products, supplies, and other frequently used items
- Clear, clean, and sufficient traffic areas

Professional Interaction

Clinical care team

Clinical care teams are often formed in healthcare facilities in order to address a patient's total wellness. Typically, a clinical care team is an interdisciplinary team comprised of various subject experts. For example, a care team may include dietary staff (manager, technician, and/or nutritionist), physicians, nurses, pharmacists, speech therapists, occupational therapists, physical therapists, social workers and/or counselors, chaplains, and/or trained volunteers. These teams meet to discuss the care plans specific to individual clients and are essential to the overall health and security of patients. A clinical care team is just one example of an interdisciplinary approach.

Interaction with different departments

A dietary manager must interact with many different departments, as the position of manager requires an individual to address all areas of an organization. Thus, a dietary manager may regularly interact with some of the following department personnel:
- Housekeeping
- Nursing/Medical
- Therapeutic
- Maintenance
- Human Resources
- Activities/Resident Development
- Facility Development (Fundraising)
- Payroll/Accounting

When interacting with personnel in and out of one's specific department, it is important that that individual be professional and respectful. A manager will inevitably communicate with other departments and organizations. It is important that all communication be done with respect for the other individual, department, and organization. Some tips for communicating effectively without individuals outside one's department include the following:
- Use introductions, including name, position, department, and organization
- Provide others with contact information, wear nametags when in person
- Promptly respond to telephone, e-mail, and postal correspondence
- Look others in the eye, shake hands firmly, take an interest in their organization/department
- Treat others with respect and dignity
- Be willing to assist others, their department and/or organization
- Respect line of authority of organization/department

Complaints are a natural occurrence in any organization. It is important that those receiving the complaints do so with dignity and respect for the client as well as the organization that they serve. First and foremost, the recipient of a complaint should always apologize for the inconvenience and/or cause of dissatisfaction and assure the client that he or she will investigate the problem further. In doing so, however, it is important that the complaint recipient assign blame or chastise any person or department to the client. Then, the complaint should be brought to the attention of the staff member's manager who may then share the concern with the appropriate department manager. Lines of authority should always be respected and observed. Complaints should be conveyed with respect, in a calm manner.

Crisis

A large crisis may never strike an organization; however a manager must be prepared in the event of a crisis. Crisis preparedness includes knowing the organization's policies and procedures for action during a crisis, to include evacuation, summoning law enforcement or ambulatory assistance, and moving staff and clients to safer areas of a facility, among others. It is important that managers take a team approach to crisis preparedness and when reacting to such an event. Roles of team members may fluctuate throughout the management of the crisis and flexibility is essential. Additionally, it is imperative that a manager to the needs of his/her clients and employees before tending to his/her own needs/desires, if possible.

Client rights

All patients and clients have rights. Some of these rights are mandated by regulating agencies, such as Centers for Medicare and Medicaid Services (CMS), the Joint Commission on Accreditation for Healthcare Organizations (JCAHO), and local and state agencies. Other rights are protected by legislation, such as HIPAA. Moreover, many facilities will draft a patient's bill of rights. Facilities and the staff working there must honor patient rights. In other words, staff must respect the wishes of the patient and adhere to policy, mandates, and legislation defining patient rights. Only when a patient is mentally incompetent may his/her wishes be overruled by an attorney-in-fact, next of kin, or other appointed individual.

Serving the community

It is important that all organizations build strong ties and healthy relationships with communities. Reaching out to a local community fosters goodwill and may present various opportunities to an organization. Ways in which a dietary department may reach out to the local community include the following:
- Provide meals to seniors
- Donate meals, supplies, or laborers to local shelters, including homeless, foster-care, domestic violence, and other shelters
- Cater local events and fundraisers
- Host civic groups, fundraisers, and other events in the organization's dining facility
- Act as an emergency shelter/soup kitchen in the event of a disaster
- Provide various health services, including screenings and education to a community
- Host dinners honoring local heroes and invite them to join residents for a meal

Business model

A business model is a plan used by an organization to research, develop, market, and execute any type of enterprise or for-profit service. A dietary manager might utilize a business model if his/her department will be offering services to a community. When developing a business model, it is important to identify the community's need and the service that will be offered to fulfill the need. Once the need is identified, it is important that the business model realistically outline the ability of the organization to execute services. This outline should include information about time, space, staffing, and financial constraints, among others. Next, the business model should identify the customer base and discuss how to market the service to the customers. Finally, the business model should project the financial implications of the service, to include cost to provide the service, associated fees, pricing (if any) of services, and profit margin, if applicable.

Local, state, and national conferences and fairs

There are many reasons why it is advisable for a manager to attend local, state, and national conferences. Conferences offer the opportunity to network, build upon skills, and refresh an organization's style. An essential aspect of business is networking. Networking is the act of meeting others in order to make mutually beneficial connections. Effective networking involves speaking with others and learning about their services and ideas. Sharing contact information is a must when networking. Conferences also offer managers the opportunity to learn new skills and approaches to various situations. These skills may be used to strengthen and refresh an organization. Moreover, conferences offer managers opportunities for personal professional development. Such development, education, and networking will make managers stronger assets to any team.

Referrals

When working with clients, it may become necessary to refer a client to another service or practitioner. It is important that a manager know when a referral is necessary and know the resources available to the client. Referrals should be noted in the medical record and may require additional written documentation. Dietary managers may have the need to refer clients to speech therapists for swallowing therapy, occupational therapists for assistance using adaptive equipment, local food delivery and senior services for clients living outside of a facility, nutritionists for personal meal plans, local support groups to help manage a disease, diet, or exercise program, or any other valuable service.

Consultation services

Consultations are a valuable aspect of providing medical care and education. Generally, consultations are made when a physician, nurse, dietitian or other health care provider would like professional advice in regards to a course of treatment. Informal consultations may be limited to verbal or written communication. Generally, however, a patient must be referred to the consultant. The consultant will then have the opportunity to evaluate the patient and report back to the consulting provider. At that point in time, it is the responsibility of the original provider to determine whether he or she will follow the course of action recommended by the consultant.
*Note: It is important to inform the patient if the consultation will incur financial obligations prior to arranging the consultation.

Client/patient confidentiality

Patients have a right to confidentiality. Therefore medical records and other documents that include identifying and sensitive information should be secured at all times. When passing information to other providers, it is important that patient confidentiality remain intact. To do this, it is important to first ensure that a referral has been made and/or a consultation has been arranged. Then, it is the responsibility of the primary provider to ensure that parties who will be receiving confidential information maintain documents in an appropriate manner. Then, confidential information should be passed in sealed documents or folders labeled "confidential."

*Note: If a patient's confidentiality is compromised, it is important that the patient be informed of the breach.

Communication with other professionals

Whether seeking the advice of a consultant, referring a patient, or networking, it is essential that communication within and outside an organization remain professional and courteous. Some tips to maintaining professional communication include the following:

- Use introductions, to include name, job title, and organization
- Make eye contact
- If possible, plan the conversation, in so far as questions and background information are involved.
- Respect other's time and opinions
- Thank others for their time and assistance

Care conferences

Care conferences are a routine part of healthcare administration. Both types of conferences, the patient-family care conference and the patient care conference, serve the needs of the patient through collaboration of individuals essential to the care of a patient or a client. A patient-family care conference is one in which the patient, his/her family and/or attorney-in-fact, and the healthcare providers are in attendance. These conferences are often scheduled to discuss the patient's care plan, a discharge, patient goals, and/or to clarify issues encountered during care. On the other hand, patient care conferences, often called care conferences, involve only the healthcare providers. The patient and his/her family are excluded from these conferences. These conferences are designed such that a team can collaborate in order to develop the most effective care plan for a specific individual.

Patient care conferences may be organized for a variety of reasons. Some of those reasons include:

- Patient/client is difficult to work with—to the point at which staff request not to serve that individual
- Patient/client's family is difficult to work with
- Lack of continuity of care
- Disagreement among providers in regards to treatment
- Treatment dilemma/questions
- Goal-setting for patient
- Pre-Patient-Family Care Conference collaboration
- Complications with current treatment plan
- Need for collaboration among multiple specialists (therapists, nutritionist or dietitian, physician, nurses, and others)

Patient-Family care conferences may be organized for a variety of reasons. Some of those reasons include:
- Discussion in regards to patient care goals
- Involving family in patient care
- Resolving conflict among patient, patient's family, and healthcare providers
- Clarifying patient and/or family treatment desires
- Referring patient to alternative services
- Lack of patient progress towards care goals
- Newly discovered illness and/or change in overall health status

Patient-family care conferences may be called to discuss positive or negative changes in the patient's health. Additionally, these conferences may be used simply as an update, as such conferences allow a discussion between the patient, his/her family, and his/her caregivers.

Because not all patient conferences are formal, documentation may not be necessary in all cases. However, it is generally advisable that meeting notes be documented and entered into the client's file. All patient-family conferences should be formally documented. Documentation should include information about who called the conference, the patient's name and name of all attendees as well as the issues that were discussed. The outcomes of the conference, to include care goals, need for future conferences, and resolution of issues, should be documented. A follow-up conference should be planned, announced, and included in the conference documentation. A copy of the documentation should be included in the patient's medical record for future reference.

Presenting a patient case

Presentation of a patient's case must be done in a thorough and professional manner. It is important that essential information be communicated in a manner that allows for discussion among collaborating professionals. Case information should include the following information about a patient:
- Age
- Sex
- Main complaint/issue
- Relevant medical/nutritional history
- Diagnosis
- Nutritional needs and goals
- Referrals to other health practitioners, community services, etc
- Treatment goals and objectives
- Issues preventing patient care and/or compliance to goals

Care planning

Care planning may be done by an individual provider or through collaboration with a team of providers. Regardless of the setting, there are some steps that should be included in every care planning process. Those steps are as follows:
1. Establish the need for care, including identification of any present illness and nutritional issues
2. Determine patient needs. These needs may extend beyond those of pure nutritional value (calorie, nutrient, and fluid intake requirements) to those of therapeutic value (swallow therapy, adaptive equipment, and/or occupational therapy).
3. Develop care goals. These goals may be nutritional, such as meeting certain caloric, nutrient, and fluid intake requirements; or, physical goals, to include the use of adaptive equipment or exercise goals. Goals must be attainable and quantifiable. Giving clients small benchmarks for which they can aim will increase motivation to work toward the greater goal.
4. Tools for meeting goals (knowledge, skills, equipment, resources)

Inspections

It is very important for a dietary manager to display professionalism during inspections, as the manager's interaction with the surveyor reflects upon the entire organization. Below are tips for being professional when working with outside inspectors/surveyors:
- Greet the inspector in a professional, respectful manner
- Ask to see inspector's identification
- Wear a nametag
- Accompany inspector on his/her tour
- Be willing and prepared to answer inspector's questions
- Always be prepared for inspection by maintaining clean, sanitary workspaces, accurate and legible records, and by doing occasional mock inspections

It is important that an organization be consistently prepared for inspection by outside organizations, as many such inspections are unannounced. In the case of announced inspections, it is advisable to review the entire department to ensure compliance with regulations, up-to-date practices and training, and to correct any lacking areas. Preparation for an inspection should include a review of previous inspections, noting and reviewing areas that may have been previously problematic. Additionally, it is advisable to carryout a "mock" inspection, in which an audit list is developed and department personnel evaluate the condition of each area of inspection. Furthermore, it is beneficial to ensure that all staff training is up-to-date and that personnel are complying with policies and procedures set forth in training. Finally, if possible, liaise with other organizations to discuss compliance issues that they have encountered. Doing so will give insight into areas under particular scrutiny by inspection teams.

Completing a self-audit is a helpful and effective way to prepare for an inspection by an outside agency. Self-audits help expose areas that are particularly weak and/or are in need of fine-tuning. Identifying and addressing problematic areas in advance of an official inspection will benefit the entire organization. To complete a self-audit, one must first identify the areas that will be scrutinized by an inspector. This can be done by obtaining a copy of the standards set forth by the regulating agency. In the event that an organization is evaluated by multiple regulatory agencies, the items evaluated by each should be consolidated into one self-audit list. Once the self-audit list is compiled, quantifiable standards should be defined for each item on the list. These standards must be written such that there is little room for varying interpretation. Once audit items are identified and measurable standards developed, the self-audit may be performed and used as a catalyst for proactive improvement.

Though inspections require detailed preparation, they should ultimately serve to improve an organization. Audits are helpful to an organization in that they are able to identify particular weaknesses of an organization's staff and facility. Moreover, inspections help to ensure the practice of health and safety standards, making the organization a better place to work as well as ensuring the health of its patrons. In many cases, audits, whether carried out by an outside regulatory agency or done as a self-audit provides an organization with valuable insight regarding problematic areas. In some cases, these problems may be identified and remedied on the spot. Other times, the inspections will identify areas for which the staff will need to brainstorm new policies and implement improved procedures in order to strengthen the organization. Finally, inspections may identify recurring problems, which, if recognized may be a catalyst for additional employee education, equipment purchase, and/or adoption of more effective practices.

Managers (and other employees) are not only allowed, but often encouraged, to ask inspectors questions in regards to regulations and compliance issues. During an inspection, an organization has the full attention of a surveyor. Thus, it is an opportune time to ask for clarification in regards to regulations, violations, and inspector comments. In the event that a manager does not understand why the facility is in violation of a regulation, it is important to ask the inspector for more information and/or ideas regarding corrective procedure while the inspector is addressing the issue. This is one of the reasons that it is important for an inspector to be escorted throughout the facility.

Corrective action may be taken in response to violations on the spot, during sanitary inspections. It is advisable to complete such action if at all possible. If the manager has questions in regards to the violation, he or she should ask the inspector for clarification when the violation is addressed. The regulating agency will dictate the degree to which immediately addressed and corrected issues must be documented. Some organizations may require a voluntary correction form as an accompaniment to the inspection form. Others may require other paperwork. The ability to immediately correct sanitary violations is one of the many reasons that inspectors should be accompanied during their audit of a facility.

An ongoing cleaning and maintenance program is essential to the upkeep of a facility, the equipment therein, and employee accountability. Therefore, such a program should assist the organization is staying inspection-ready throughout daily operations. Ongoing cleaning and maintenance programs require employee accountability, in that employees are assigned cleaning and/or maintenance duties and must perform those duties on a preset schedule. The duties are performed on some sort of rotation schedule, which promotes teamwork and additional accountability. Moreover, such programs may assist in the identification of problem areas and the need for employee education.

Production, Safety, and Business Management

Manage Supplies, Sanitation & Safety

Critical control point

A critical control point (CCP) is a limit set in order to ensure food safety. At this limit, controls can be applied such that food hazards are eliminated and/or are reduced to a level within the acceptable parameters. The most common application of critical control points is in cooking, where temperatures are assigned to determine safety of various foods. Those measures, when taken at the thickest part of a meat are as follows:

- 135° -- Cooked fruits, vegetables, and any commercially processed food that will be held for an extended period before being consumed
- 145° -- Roasts, steaks, chops, fish, eggs
- 155° -- Ground meats or fish, injected meats, eggs that will not be immediately consumed
- 165° -- Poultry, stuffing, stuffed items (including meats, fish, pasta, and poultry), any food that was allowed to cool and/or was refrigerated and that will be reheated from a temperature below 135°

**Note: Temperatures must be sustained for varying amounts of time, usually ranging from 4-15 seconds.

Hazard Analysis Critical Control Point

The following are the seven principles of Hazard Analysis Critical Control Point (HACCP):

- Principle 1: Conduct a hazard analysis in which any food safety hazard, such as those presented by chemical, biological or physical composition and/or properties is determined
- Principle 2: Determine critical control points by setting limits which serve to eliminate and/or reduce any potential food risk
- Principle 3: Develop preventative measures, to include critical limits, for each critical control point
- Principle 4: Institute critical control point monitoring procedures. These monitoring procedures and the frequency with which they are carried out must be listed in the HACCP plan.
- Principle 5: Develop corrective actions which will rectify any situation in which the monitoring procedures show that critical limits have not been reached
- Principle 6: Verify that all procedures as well as the HACCP system are correctly working
- Principle 7: Institute an efficient data system to document and maintain HACCP system records

Hazard Analysis Critical Control Point records should include the following information:
- An analysis summary which outlines and justifies the hazards and control points
- The HACCP plan, including information about the team and responsibilities of each individual, description of food and services to the consumer, a flow diagram of the process, and a plan summary. The plan summary should incorporate each of the seven principles (critical control points, critical limits, applicable hazards, monitoring, corrective actions, verification, and records log).
- Supporting documentation
- Information logged during the implementation of the plan

Capital equipment

Capital equipment is defined as equipment essential to the function of a job that is usually characterized by an expensive price tag and a long life. So, for example, an appliance such as a meat slicer, refrigerator, or microwave may be classified as capital equipment. Each facility should define "expensive;" some organizations define items priced at $500 or more capital equipment, while others put a higher or lower price on capital equipment. Regardless of the organization's price definition, capital equipment typically needs to be approved before purchase. The process of purchasing such equipment should include: establishing a need, determining whether money is available in the budget, shop for vendors, models, and prices, ask for the opinions of others within the organization, and prepare a document justifying the purchase. Then, the financial offer can make an informed decision in regards to purchasing the item.

Equipment vendors

There are many different ways to find equipment vendors, and it is important to shop around, especially when making capital equipment purchases. Some vendors may offer discounts for multiple sales, a large scale, or to specific organizations. Discounts may also be offered to organizations that frequently buy from a specific vendor. When shopping for equipment, it is often helpful to examine and use the equipment in person as well as read the specifications. Therefore, it is advisable to visit local supplies and trade shows to view sample items. Before buying, however, check the catalogs and websites of other vendors. When buying, compare price against specifications and warranty. Some vendors will add extended warranties to their product for an additional cost.

Equipment specification

Information compiled for an equipment specification includes the following:
- Name
- Dimensions
- Capacity
- Energy and/or power needs
- Warranty
- Delivery requirements
- Approval/Certifications needed
- Training Requirements
- Interior and exterior construction materials

- Additional features and/or accessories needed
- Compatibility with available space, kitchen design, and other equipment
- Ability to fulfill the current and projected needs of the organization

Preventative maintenance

Preventative maintenance is a schedule of cleaning, fixing, and tuning-up equipment to increase its life. It is important that all equipment, especially capital equipment undergo routine preventative maintenance and inspections to ensure the item is operating properly and safely. Though preventative maintenance may seem to be a hassle, it prevents serious inconvenience in the long-term. Preventative maintenance increases the life of a product, reduces costs associated with fixing and replacing the item, ensures employee safety, and maximizes the organization's resources. The unanticipated failure of equipment may lead to more labor costs as the organization attempts to purchase additional equipment.

USDA inspection

The United States Department of Agriculture (USDA) mandates that certain most meat and poultry products be inspected by the Food Safety and Inspection Service (FSIS). These inspections are designed to ensure that the food is safe for consumption, of "wholesome" quality, and is labeled correctly before being passed to consumers. The FSIS inspects all meat and poultry products being sold in the United States, whether they originate from foreign or domestic sources. Once food is inspected and approved, the meat carcass is stamped with an inspection seal. Certain meats, such as popular game (deer, elk, antelope, buffalo, and rabbit, among others), do not require a federal inspection. However, a voluntary inspection may be requested (and paid for) by businesses.

USDA grading

The United States Department of Agriculture (USDA) offers a voluntary service to meat producers and processors called grading. Grading is done by a Federal grader, who evaluates the qualities of meat. The grader will assign a grade based upon the meat's texture, quality, perceived taste, tenderness, and other similar factors. Poultry is also evaluated based on shape and fullness of meat. Each grade requires that certain, federal standards are met. These criteria ensure that meat and poultry products are consistently evaluated, regardless of the inspector. Poultry and meat product packages will display the grade. Grading is a voluntary service, and therefore, producers must pay to have their products graded.

Meat products are evaluated using two types of grades. The first of those grades is a quality grade. The quality grade represents the perceived quality of meat, incorporating the meat's tenderness, flavor, and juiciness. Quality beef grades include: prime, choice, select, standard, commercial, utility, cutter, and canner. The second type of meat grade is a yield grade. The yield grade denotes the amount of "usable" meat on a carcass. Yield grades range from one to five, with one being the highest and five the lowest grade. Consumers may not find yield grades particularly valuable except when buying very large cuts of meat.

There are eight grades of beef. Those grades are as follows:
- Prime: Originates from young, healthy cattle. Typically served in restaurants. Flavorful and characterized by lots of marbling.
- Choice: Includes very tender cuts as well as some that are less tender and are more easily over-cooked using dry-heat. Less marbling than prime cuts.
- Select: Often leaner than the higher grade; therefore, select grades are often best prepared by marinating
- Standard/Commercial: Less tender and flavorful. May not be labeled as graded.
- Utility/Cutter/Canner: Often used in processed products

Veal, lamb, and pork grades differ in standard as well as number of grades. There are five grades for veal. Those grades include prime, choice, good, standard, and utility. Typically, veal sold at retail stores is graded at the prime or choice level. Lamb is also graded with five grades, prime, choice, good, utility, and cull. Typically, only lamb graded as prime or choice are offered in retail markets. Remember, the higher the grade of meat, the more flavorful, juicy, and tender the meat will be. These characteristics directly result from the amount of marbling in the meat. When choosing lower grades of meat, it is advisable to pick more tender cuts. Pork is not graded by the USDA.

Poultry is assigned three grades by the United States Department of Agriculture (USDA). Those grades are A, B, and C. Grade A is the most commonly seen grade of poultry in retail stores. These pieces are generally intact and do not exhibit any discolorations, feathers, or other defects. Grade A poultry that is not skinned, will have intact skin, and the appearance of the flesh will be full and plump. Bones will not be broken in bone-in products. Poultry graded B and C are often used in processed foods and are rarely sold intact. Certain parts of poultry are not graded. Those parts include the neck, wing tips, tails, and giblets.

Potable water and the Safe Drinking Water Act

Potable water is any water that is deemed safe to drink and free from contamination. Water is labeled as "potable" even in the cases where it may not be used for drinking but is safe enough to be used for that purpose. The Safe Drinking Water Act is the primary law regulating water safety in the United States. The law was enacted in 1974, and is meant to protect Americans by protecting water sources. Essentially, the act allows the Environmental Protection Agency (EPA) to set certain standards for drinking water. The EPA then works with public water sources to ensure that the standards are met and maintained and that all drinking water is free of harmful contaminates.

Obtaining safe drinking water

Because all public sources of drinking water are regulated by the Safe Drinking Water Act and the Environmental Protection Agency (EPA), managers can rest assured water, labeled as potable, from approved public sources is safe to cook with and/or serve to clients. Additionally, private or commercial water sources meeting the standards set forth by the EPA and the Safe Drinking Water Act are safe to cook with and serve. Water from private sources should be annually tested, at minimum. If utilizing a private water vendor, it is advisable to request a copy of the organization's consumer confidence report and any additional test results.

Purchasing seafood

As with other types of food, it is important that seafood, including fish and shellfish be purchased from an approved, regulated vendor. Buying outside of regulated vendors may put customers at risk of contamination and illness and, therefore, may jeopardize the health and reputation of an organization. Seafood, like other foods, is regulated by the United States Food and Drug Administration. The FDA has paired with other nation's food safety agencies to evaluate and approve certain shellfish vendors. Those vendor's names are included on the Interstate Certified Shellfish Shippers List. Buyers may purchase shellfish (edible pieces of oysters, clams, mussels, and scallops) with confidence from these vendors. Many states also have regulations governing seafood distribution with respective vendor lists. These may also serve as a resource for safe seafood purchase.

According to the United States Food and Drug Administration (US FDA), the following characteristics generally indicate seafood freshness:
- Mild smell, not overly fishy or ammonia-like
- Clear, slightly bulging eyes, not sunken or cloudy
- Skin that is firm and shiny
- Bright red gills, free from slime
- Springy flesh
- Fillets that are free from discoloration (brown, yellow, or green) do not appear mushy, dry, or dark

When buying frozen fish, be sure that the package is fully sealed and free from holes and sits lower in the store's freezer. Additionally, if the fish is visible through the package, avoid buying fish that has a dry appearance and/or is covered with frost or ice.

Graded eggs

Not all eggs and egg products are graded by the United States Department of Agriculture (USDA). Egg producers and packers may voluntarily submit to USDA grading, which ensures that their products conform to the highest standards. Other egg and egg product producers are subject to state regulation. When purchasing eggs for commercial use, it is important to select eggs that have been graded by the USDA - preferably, grade AA or A. Though the highly graded eggs may be more expensive than eggs offered by other vendors, the organization has quality assurance. Buying "farm-fresh," ungraded eggs is not recommended. The USDA assigns three grades to eggs; those grades are AA, A, and B. Grades are assigned based upon the eggshell appearance and the interior quality of the egg. Eggs of the same grade may differ in size.

The qualities denoted by each grade are listed below:
- US Grade AA: Thick, firm egg whites; round, high, nearly perfect yolks; clean, unbroken shells
- US Grade A: "Reasonably firm" egg whites; high, round yolks, generally free of defects; clean, unbroken shells
- US Grade B: Thinner egg whites; wide, somewhat flat yolks; eggshell may have visible stains

Generally, retailers carry US Grade A eggs.

Organic foods

Recent years have seen a shift in food production in which growers are producing and marketing "organic" foods. Organic foods are those that are grown without the use of pesticides, synthesized fertilizers, and without exposure to human waste or sewage. Animal products that are certified organic are not typically injected with growth hormone or antibiotics. Additionally, many of the animals are raised on organic feed and do not have any genetic modifications. In the United States, the United States Department of Agriculture has adopted the National Organic Program which certifies organic foods based upon the standards set forth by that program.

Food storage and temperature

It is important that food shipments/purchases be tested for proper temperature before signing in receipt of the goods. Food delivered at temperatures above that at which they should be stored is susceptible to spoilage. In the case of such a delivery, the food from that delivery should be thrown out. Poultry, seafood, meat, and egg products should all be received at or below 41°F if refrigerated and below 0°F if frozen. Dairy products should be received at a temperature between 6°F and 10°F, if frozen. Otherwise, dairy products should be refrigerated below 41°F.

Time/temperature indicators (TTI) strips are also known as shelf-life indicators. These strips change color to indicate whether a product is still considered fresh or safe. The indicator is programmed to change when a product reaches its expiration date or if it has been stored incorrectly, thus resulting in the possibility of spoilage. The TTI strip should be examined when receiving goods and any products with a changed strip should be rejected and disposed of properly. Never serve or use products whose indicator strips have changed color, as it poses unnecessary risk to consumers.

It is important to assign shipment receiving to a trained employee, as the incoming food must be checked for quality assurance purposes. Food that does not meet the quality and safety standards of an organization should not be accepted from the vendor, and a refund should be immediately requested. The following is a list of quality indicators that should be checked during receipt of a shipment:
- Temperature of potentially hazardous foods (PHF/TCS)
- Packaging. Reject products with defective, suspect, or tampered packaging
- Inspection stamps and dates
- Food expiration and/or use-by dates
- Quality of food, to include color, texture, and odor

Meat storage
It is important to properly store all food products to ensure that the items do not become susceptible to foodborne pathogens that may cause illness to clients. Additionally, taste and texture of foods deteriorate with the item's shelf-life. If stored at the correct temperatures, which are 0°F for frozen meats and at or below 41°F, beef may be stored in the freezer for approximately 6-12 months. Refrigerated beef should be used within 3-6 days of purchase. Ground beef should only be stored for 3-4 months in the freezer and up to 2 days in the refrigerator. If upon, thawing, evidence of freezer burn, discoloration, or odor is present, it is best to dispose of the beef entirely.

Poultry and egg storage

It is important to properly store all food products to ensure that the items do not become susceptible to foodborne pathogens that may cause illness to clients. Additionally, taste and texture of foods deteriorate with the item's shelf-life. Poultry and egg products should be refrigerated at a temperature no greater than 41°F and should be frozen at or below 0°F. Poultry has a shelf-life of approximately 6 months when stored in a freezer but should be used within a couple of days if refrigerated. Eggs and egg products shelf-life differ, based on the type of product. Generally speaking, fresh eggs should be used within 1-2 weeks of purchase. For egg products that are packed or in a carton, check the use by label on the carton for guidance.

Seafood storage

It is important to properly store all food products to ensure that the items do not become susceptible to foodborne pathogens that may cause illness to clients. Additionally, taste and texture of foods deteriorate with the item's shelf-life. Seafood products may last as long as 4 months when properly stored in a freezer at a temperature no higher than 0°F. If refrigerated, at a temperature at or below 41°F, seafood products are safe to prepare up to two days after the date of purchase. Do not prepare seafood that appears discolored, freezer-burned, or has a particularly fishy odor. Seafood in that condition should be disposed of immediately.

Dairy storage

It is important to properly store all food products to ensure that the items do not become susceptible to foodborne pathogens that may cause illness to clients. Additionally, taste and texture of foods deteriorate with the item's shelf-life. Dairy products have a wide range of shelf-lives depending upon whether the item is pasteurized, processed, and the type of product. Always use the expiration date on the carton or packaging as a guide for using and disposing dairy products. Generally speaking, dairy products should be stored at a maximum temperature of 41°F in the refrigerator and a maximum temperature of 0°F in the freezer. Some dairy products packaged in UHT packaging may be stored at room temperature, if the package remains unopened.

General food storage guidelines

Food must not only be stored at proper temperatures, but in an orderly fashion that prevents contamination of food by humans, other foods, and pests. Therefore the following guidelines apply to food storage:
- Store food on shelves that are at least 6" from the ground
- Store food away from walls and ceilings
- Store food in containers that protect products from contamination or infestation
- Store food in such a way to avoid cross-contamination
- Sort and store meat and poultry products by type
- Store pre-cooked and ready-to-eat foods above raw meats, poultry, seafood, etc., to avoid contamination from leaking juices
- Store food away from chemicals, cleansers, leaks, and any other source of contamination
- Do not store food in restrooms, changing areas, stairwells, or any other area that may be contaminated by human waste and germs
- Store food in a well-ventilated, cool, dry area

Shelf-life of basic staples

Every food product has a shelf-life. Taste and texture of foods deteriorate with time, and many foods may spoil, leading to a health hazard for consumers. Look to the food packaging for specific dates regarding shelf-life. Below are some general guidelines in regards to shelf life:

- Baking powder: 18 months
- Baking soda: 2 years
- Chocolate: 18 months
- Coffee can, unopened: 2 years
- Corn Syrup: 3 years
- Cornstarch: 18 months
- Flour: 6-8 months
- Honey: 12 months
- Rice, white: 2 years
- Rice, brown: 6-12 months
- Shortening: 8 months
- Sugar, granulated: 2 years
- Sugar, brown: 4 months
- Vinegar, unopened: 2 years

Date labels

Many food products are labeled with a date. That date may be a "sell by," "expiration," "use by," or "packed on" date. It is important to understand the definition of these terms so that food is properly stored, used, and disposed of when necessary. The terms are defined below:

- Sell by dates note the last date by which a product should be sold from the retailer. These dates allow consumers a period of a few days past the designated date to use the product.
- Expiration dates note the last day that a food product should be consumed or used for cooking. It is prudent to dispose of food that has past its expiration date.
- Use by dates are a sort of quality assurance, in that these dates note the date on which the product may start loosing its freshness
- Packed on dates note the day on which a food was canned, packaged, and/or processed

Appropriate storage temperatures

Appropriate storage temperatures are as follows:

- Freezer: 0°F, maximum
- Deep Chill: 26°F-32°F
- Refrigerator: 41°F, maximum
- Dry Storage: 50-70°F

It is important that foods be stored at (or in the case of freezer and refrigerator storage, below) their respective storage temperatures to maintain the integrity of the product. Storing food above the designated temperature introduces the risk of spoilage and contamination. It is particularly dangerous to allow food needing refrigeration to sit at a temperature between 40°F-140°F, as it is in this range that it is easiest for bacteria to grow and multiply.

FIFO

FIFO is the acronym for "First In, First Out." The "first in, first out" principle is a guideline for using, moving, and handling food. When an organization receives a delivery of food, the older products should be rotated to the front of the shelf, and the new products placed behind the older products. When the food stores are rotated in this manner, it ensures that food is used in the order it is received, thus minimizing food waste. Even with proper rotation, it is important that food dates always be checked prior to using and/or serving food products to ensure that the food is still safe for consumption.

Packaging

Food packaging compromises
The quality of packaged food may be compromised when the packaging is disturbed, torn, dented, or defective in anyway. When receiving food purchases, it is important to check all packaging for flaws and disturbance. Be particularly vigilant of packages that show evidence of dents, rust, tears, leaks, or other damage and/or tampering. These products should be rejected at delivery or disposed of if the damage occurs between delivery and use. Additionally, eggs that are delivered with cracked or discolored shells should also be discarded. It is never prudent to prepare meals using food from damaged containers.

Modified atmosphere packaging and controlled atmosphere packaging
In an effort to extend the shelf-life of various foods, food manufacturers have developed processes that result in modified atmosphere packaging (MAP) and/or controlled atmosphere packaging (CAP). Such packaging uses a variation of atmospheric gases in order to stunt the deterioration of food. In most cases, the level of oxygen in a package is significantly reduced, sometimes until oxygen is no longer present. Other gases occupy the airy space of a package. While these methods may prevent visible spoilage of foods, MAP and CAP packaging does not prevent contamination of food by anaerobic microbes.

Ultra-pasteurization and ultra-high temperature packaging
Ultra-pasteurization is a food processing option that uses extremely high heat, of at least 280°F, for a short period of time, generally a matter of seconds, to kill microorganisms and harmful bacteria in food. This process is effective in prolonging the shelf-life of foods; however, it does not eliminate the need for refrigeration. Some ultra-pasteurized foods are also packaged in ultra-high temperature (UHT) packaging. UHT packaging is aseptic. As a result, foods that are processed through ultra-pasteurization and ultra-high temperature packaging do not ultimately require refrigeration and are considered stable for shelf storage.

Selecting a food vendor

Food vendors abound, and it is, therefore, important to carefully select vendors from which to order an organization's food supplies. A vendor must be reliable in all regards, including food quality and safety, prompt and courteous delivery, reasonable prices, etc. Below are some things to consider when selecting a food vendor:
- Quality of vendor's products and service
- Willingness to schedule convenient deliveries for organization
- Willingness to have all deliveries inspected

- Willingness to refund monies for food rejected at delivery
- Quality of vendor's equipment, to include storage facility/warehouse, delivery trucks, refrigerator/freezer equipment
- Vendor's reputation and record of service
- Follows a HACCP process
- Subjects itself to inspection and willing to present inspection findings to customers

Foodborne illness

Foodborne illness is any type of disease or pathogen that is transmitted by food or food products. Foodborne illness most often manifests with "flu-like" symptoms, to include diarrhea, vomiting, fever, headache, chills, and others, though it may take on other symptoms. In severe cases, foodborne illness may lead to death. These types of illnesses are not transferable from one person to another, as the cause of the illness is linked to consumed food. When two or more people contract a foodborne illness from the same food, and chemical analyses confirm that the food was the culprit of the illness, a foodborne illness "outbreak" is declared.

Foodborne illness is caused by a variety of contaminating factors. Those factors are divided into three broad categories: biological pathogens, chemical hazards, and physical contaminants. Biological pathogens include: bacteria (including e coli), viruses, parasites, natural toxins, fungi, and prions. Chemical hazards include contamination by cleaning supplies, pesticides sprayed on crops, and materials used during production, manufacturing, and packaging. Physical contaminants include dirt, body/animal hair, bone, shards of plastic, metal, glass, wood, rocks and other materials.

Bacteria in canned goods

There are many types of bacteria and these bacteria grow under a variety of conditions. For example, aerobic bacteria must have exposure to oxygen to live and grown whereas anaerobic bacteria do not have that need. Some bacteria can grow with or without oxygen, those types are called facultative. Therefore, it is possible for bacteria to grow, even in canned goods or from the center of foods. The danger of bacterial growth and/or bacteria-released toxins is much higher when food packaging is damaged; therefore, it is important to reject all items with packaging defects.

Bacteria growing conditions

Bacteria are microorganisms, and as such, it requires certain conditions to grow. Those conditions include:
- Appropriate temperature. The typical danger zone for bacterial growth is between 41°F -135°F
- Presence of oxygen, depending upon the type of bacteria
- Time exposure. It is best not to serve food that has been in the "danger zone" for an extended period of time (between 2-4 hours)
- Moisture
- pH of food; bacteria is more likely to grow in slightly acidic conditions
- Nutrient composition

Common bacterial pathogens

There are many types of foodborne bacterial pathogens. Some of the most commonly encountered pathogens include:
- Aeromonas hydrophilia
- Bacillus cereus
- Campylobacter jejuni
- Clostridium botulinum
- Clostridium perfringens
- Listeria monocytogenes
- Salmonella enteritidis
- Shiga Toxin-Producing Escherichia coli
- Shigella
- Staphylococcus aureus
- Vibrio cholerae
- Vibrio parahaemolyticus
- Yersinia enterocolitica

Fatalities

Foodborne illnesses may, in fact, be fatal if not properly detected or treated. While most foodborne illness will pass within a matter of hours or days, some illness can be so severely dehydrating and/or may attack one's immune system in a fatal manner. Typical symptoms of foodborne illness include nausea, vomiting, diarrhea, muscle pain, fever, abdominal pain, difficulties swallowing, breathing, or speaking, headache, chills, cramping, and dehydration. Illness onset may be anywhere from one hour to a matter of days, depending upon the type of pathogen. All foodborne illnesses should be reported.

Foodborne viruses

Viruses that are contracted from the consumption of food are often classified as gastroenteritis viruses. These viruses most often cause symptoms such as nausea, vomiting, diarrhea, and abdominal cramping. Foodborne viruses are generally spread from person-to-person, in that an infected food service worker may contaminate foods later consumed by a customer. Additionally, certain foods, namely seafood, can carry viruses. While viruses are life forms, they do not grow on or in foods. Some of the most common foodborne viruses include:
- Hepatitis A
- Hepatitis E
- Norovirus
- Rotavirus

Foodborne parasites

Parasites are organisms that live and feed off of a "host," which is another living organism. Foodborne parasites include worms, insects, and protozoa. Parasites are most commonly found in meat and seafood, though they may be present on fruits and vegetables as well as in milk and water. Common symptoms of parasites include muscle pain, abdominal cramping, fever, diarrhea, bloating, weight loss, and symptoms of malnourishment as the body is not given the opportunity to absorb important vitamins, minerals, and nutrients.

Commonly identified foodborne parasites include:
- Acanthamoeba
- Anisakis
- Ascaris lumbricoides
- Cryptosporidium parvum
- Cyclospora cayetanensis
- Diphyllobothrium
- Entamoeba histolytica
- Giardia lamblia
- Nanophyetus
- Trichinella spiralis
- Trichuris trichiura

Foodborne fungi

Fungus is most often present in foods in the forms of mold or yeast. Sometimes, therefore, fungus is helpful in producing foods, such as the production of yeast-breads and cheeses (mold). However, these types of fungi may also be hazardous, in that they can release toxins called mycotoxins. The types of mycotoxins that commonly appear in food include: aflatoxins, deoxynivalenol, fumonisin, nivalenol, ochratoxin A, and zearalenone. Mycotoxins may lead to serious neurological problems, and several mycotoxins are suspected to be carcinogens. Mold typically appears as a dark greenish-black, fuzzy growth on the surface of food. Most fungi, in particular mold spores, need three things to grow: moisture, time, and some sort of nutrient, generally of organic material. Yeast may spoil food through a process of fermentation, which may be detected by food discoloration or an alcohol-like odor. Many foods may be safely consumed, even if mold is present on the product. It is important, however, to cut away the moldy part of the food as well as a one inch section of the food surrounding the mold. Mold may be removed from the following items, which can later be safely served:
- Apples
- Bell peppers
- Broccoli
- Brussel Sprouts
- Cabbage
- Cauliflower
- Firm cheeses, i.e., Swiss, cheddar
- Garlic
- Onions
- Pears
- Potatoes
- Turnips
- Winter Squash
- Zucchini

*Note: Cheeses that are intentionally moldy, such as blue, gorgonzola, and stilton varieties may be consumed without cutting out the visible mold.

Prions

Prions are pathogens that are entirely comprised of damaged or mutated proteins. These pathogens attack the neurological system of animals and humans. The neurodegenesis is untreatable and fatal. Prions are responsible for "mad-cow disease," bovine spongiform encephalopathy. Prions are responsible for Creutzfeldt-Jakob disease, Gerstmann-Strauussler-Scheinker syndrome, fatal familial insomnia, sporadic fatal insomnia, Kuru, and Alpers syndrome. Prions are only infectious when one consumed as part of an animal source. Prion infection is highly unlikely, though risk does exist. The greatest risk of infection by prions occurs when bovine neural tissue (brain, spinal cord, nerves) and/or parts of the small intestines are consumed.

Natural toxins

Toxins naturally occur in some plants and animals. Natural toxins are most commonly found in seafood and mushrooms. Often times, toxins in seafood develop after the sea animal eats from algae. Naturally occurring toxins may also be present in red beans and honey. Symptoms resulting from illness caused by natural toxins are primarily neurological though it is not uncommon to experience gastrointestinal symptoms such as vomiting, diarrhea, and abdominal cramping. Some natural toxins also affect the human cardiovascular system. The most effective way to avoid naturally occurring toxins is to buy seafood and mushrooms from reliable, approved, and inspected sources.

Highly susceptible populations

Highly susceptible populations are those in which there is a greater risk of contracting an illness or experiencing the illness and its symptoms more severely than in normal populations. Children, the elderly, pregnant women, and individuals with suppressed immune system functioning are all considered highly susceptible populations. These populations are not only more likely to experience more severe symptoms of foodborne illness but the peripheral effects, such as malabsorption of nutrients and dehydration are more drastic, and therefore, more difficult to recover from than in a healthy adult. Accordingly, the Food and Drug Administration (FDA) stipulates that greater care must be taken when serving these populations in order to protect them from foodborne illness.

Cross-contamination

Cross-contamination is the transfer of pathogens from any item to food during the production, preparation, and service of food items. Cross-contamination is a major cause of foodborne illness and should be avoided. Food can easily be contaminated by coming in contact with other foods, contaminated equipment, or an individual who is carrying a pathogen. Cross-contamination often occurs when equipment is not properly cleaned between uses and/or the food service worker does not follow correct hand-washing and handling procedure. Additionally, cross-contamination is likely to occur when unwashed produce or raw meats come in contact with clean, ready to eat foods.

Cross-contamination may be prevented by following some simple guidelines. Those include:

- Thoroughly wash hands between handling food, after using the restroom and/or performing any personal grooming
- Store cooked and raw foods separate from one another. Never store raw foods above cooked foods, to avoid spillage of juices.
- Do not use the same cutting board and knife to cut cooked foods as was used for raw foods
- Thoroughly wash and sanitize all utensils and equipment that comes in contact with food
- Keep washed and unwashed foods away from one another

Proper thawing techniques

Food should never be thawed on a kitchen counter. Doing so allows the food to sit in the "hazard" zone for a lengthy amount of time, putting the item at risk for bacterial growth and foodborne pathogens. Rather, food should be thawed in the refrigerator, at a temperature no greater than 41°F. Food may also be thawed by placing it in an airtight, water-tight plastic bag, and submerged in cold water. The water should remain running or should, at least, be changed every 20 minutes. In some cases, food may be thawed in the oven during cooking. Generally, frozen foods will take at least 1.5 times as long as those already thawed to cook. Finally, food may be thawed completely in a microwave. Use this method only if the food will be cooked entirely immediately after thawing.

Monitoring food temperature

It is important to know how to measure food temperatures accurately, as a food thermometer may be the most effective tool in warning that food may be subject to foodborne illness. To correctly measure food temperature, it is important to use a food thermometer. Insert the thermometer into the center and/or thickest part of the food item, being careful to avoid touching bone, fat, or any part of the pan. In the case of frozen items, a thermometer may be inserted between frozen packages of food. Regardless of whether the temperature of hot or cold foods is being measured, it is important to leave the thermometer in place for several seconds to ensure an accurate reading. Finally, the thermometer must be thoroughly washed and sanitized between uses.

It is important that foods be heated to an appropriate endpoint temperature. To ensure that foods reach the endpoint temperature, one should measure the internal temperature of a food with a food thermometer. Typically a bi-metallic stem thermometer is used to measure the internal temperature of larger portions of food. These thermometers generally require that a fairly large surface area, close to 3" of the probe be in contact with the interior portion of the food being measured. When a large measuring surface area is not available, it is important to use a smaller-diameter probe, such as a thermistor or thermocouple thermometer.

Hot foods must be maintained at a temperature of at least 135ºF (140 ºF, according to some sources). Food may be kept at this temperature by using warming plates, steaming tables, and other specialized equipment. When holding and transporting food, it is important that foods maintain a healthy and safe temperature. Thus, it is imperative that temperature be measured frequently, at least every two hours. If the temperature falls below a safe measurement, the food should be immediately reheated or discarded. In the case of buffet or trayline service, it is also recommended that an entire pan of food act as a refill. In other words, fresh, hot food should not be poured onto food that has been sitting.

As with hot holding, cold holding is regulated by the food temperature. Foods should stay at or below a temperature of 41 ºF, to maintain the safety and integrity of the food. Food may be transported in refrigerator units or may be placed in ice baths, excepted when packaging may allow water or ice to come into direct contact with the food. Generally speaking, unpackaged foods may not come into contact with undrained iced. Again, it is imperative that temperatures be regularly monitored and logged to ensure the safety of foods. During food service, utensils may be in contact with the food, however, between uses, the utensils should be stored in water that is at least 135 ºF.

Leftovers

If leftover food is handled correctly, it may be served again. Follow these tips for storing, reheating, and serving leftovers:
- Discard food that has been at room temperature for more than two hours
- Quick-chill or separate food into small containers to cool before placing in the refrigerator
- Refrigerate leftovers immediately (or once cooled by quick-chilling/dividing into smaller containers)
- Reheat leftovers to at least 165°F before serving
- Do not reheat leftovers more than once. Discard remaining leftovers after first reheating.
- If leftovers have been frozen, thaw in the refrigerator or while cooking
- Do not keep leftovers for more than 7 days, if stored in a refrigerator

Slacking

According to the FDA Food Code, slacking is "the process of moderating the temperature of a food" in order to properly prepare an item, so that the product retains taste, texture, and safety quality. Slacking is most often used to bring frozen foods to an appropriate temperature before deep fat frying. Additionally, slacking may be used to bring foods that are frozen in blocks to a temperature that more readily facilitates even heating. When slacking foods from frozen to ready-to-cook, it is important that the temperature of the food not exceed 41°F. Allowing foods to slack beyond that point may make them susceptible to spoilage and/or contamination.

Special attention for highly susceptible populations

The FDA Food Code mandates that eggs, juices, and fresh seed sprouts must be handled with additional care. The FDA Food Code prohibits serving eggs that are not fully cooked to highly susceptible populations. This regulation applies to meringues, soufflés, soft-cooked eggs, raw eggs, among others. Additionally, it is highly recommended that that treated egg products or pasteurized eggs be used for any recipe in which more than one egg is called for. Juices must also be processed or pasteurized before serving to highly susceptible populations. Fresh seed sprouts and raw meats are strictly prohibited by the Food Code for service to these populations.

Date marking

Date marking is used to indicate the date by which a food should consumed, used, or disposed. Date marking applies to potentially hazardous foods (PHF/TCS) as well as to leftovers. As with all other foods, these items should be stored at or below a temperature of 41 ºF. If this temperature is exceeded, the item should be immediately disposed of. All foods should be disposed of in seven days (with the day the food was opened being day one) if they have not been consumed. There are certain exceptions to the date marking rule; those include: semi-soft and hard cheeses, uncut portions of processed, cured meats, and commercially acidified dressings.

Food service regulatory agencies

Food service is regulated by many agencies. It is important that a facility be in compliance with all applicable regulatory agencies, as noncompliance may result in fines, illness, and even closing of the facility. The following are some of the many agencies that may regulate food service operations:
- Local government
- State government
- Federal government
- Food and Drug Administration (FDA)
- United States Department of Agriculture (USDA)
- Centers for Disease Control and Prevention (CDC)
- National Marine Fisheries Service (NMFS)

Crisis

A crisis is a sudden, generally unexpected, change. This change may occur on any level, to include personal, organizational, societal, or environmental. Crises may often be managed but are not always preventable. Types of crises that a food service organization may encounter include:
- Flood
- Tornado
- Tropical Storm
- Fire
- Earthquake
- Illness of employee or customer
- Employee strike
- Vendor strike
- Food tampering
- Food contamination
- Violence
- Foodborne illness
- Public works (utility) dysfunction
- Terrorism
- Food Shortage
- Public protesting

Food service organizations should prepare for crises and emergency situations. Certain organizations, such as hospitals, long-term care facilities, and other institutions responsible for the care of individuals must have an emergency plan. That plan may include the following:
- Stocking bottled water, canned goods, and disposable dinnerware
- Preparing an emergency menu, utilizing canned good stockpile
- Developing fire, earthquake, and tornado evacuation plans
- Posting the contact information for local emergency services
- Posted plans for handing bomb, bioterrorism, and violent threats
- Management of a foodborne illness outbreak, including instructions regarding media inquiries

Bioterrorism

It is important that every link in the "farm-to-table chain" actively work to prevent bioterrorism, as the impact of a successfully carried out attack is widespread. Such an event may touch a vast population before being neutralized, which may lead to unnecessary fatalities, tremendous healthcare costs, economic concerns, and an agricultural crisis. Prevention techniques include the following:
- Perform a vulnerability assessment
- Routinely make security of checks, especially of vulnerable areas
- Encourage employees to report suspicious activities
- Implement identification badge security
- Limit access to vulnerable areas, including storage, mixing, etc.
- Prohibit off-duty employee access to food service and production areas
- Report any concerns

According to the FDA, food tampering may occur at any level of the food production chain. That is to say, a threat may be introduced during the cultivation of crops and livestock, distribution, processing, manufacturing, sell, delivery, storage, preparation, or service of the foodstuffs. Food is vulnerable to tampering during any phase of this chain and should tampering occur, the results could be devastating. Therefore, it is important to implement security procedures to minimize the likelihood for tampering. Food security has risen to a level of concern so high that it has been included in the Bioterrorism Act of 2002.

There are many characteristics of food which make the product attractive to bioterrorists. According to the FDA, some of those characteristics include production of large batches, uniform mixing of items, short shelf life, and easy access to the food. Foodstuffs with these attributes provide a bioterrorist with the opportunity to quickly and efficiently taint a large quantity of food and/or carry out an act that may be difficult to detect and contain because of the short amount of time in which a product is sold and consumed. Moreover, foods with vibrant flavors, colors, or odors are also attractive targets for bioterrorists as they may more easily conceal a contaminant.

Any food security concerns should be reported immediately. It is important that this be emphasized to all employees, and the staff should be encouraged to error on the side of caution. In the event of suspected food tampering, the local law enforcement authority should be immediately contacted for investigation. Next, the FDA Office of Emergency Operations and/or the Food Safety and Inspection Service Office of Food Security and

Emergency Preparedness should be contacted on their 24-hour hotline. In the event that it appears livestock has been tampered with, the Animal and Plant Health Inspection Service should also be notified.

Food safety and food security

While both food safety and food security are used in reference to maintaining the integrity and quality of food, as well as consumer safety, these terms are not equivalent. Food safety is the term applied to measures and processes which are implemented in order to protect food from unintentional contamination, such as contamination as a result of naturally pathogens or by poor food handling practices. On the other hand, food security is the term used in reference to protecting food from intentional acts of tampering and contamination, such as bioterrorist threats, during any part of the "farm-to-table-chain."

Corrective action

A corrective action is the action that is taken in order to meet the requirements of a critical limit (physical, chemical or biological characteristic of food which may be used as an indicator of a hazard). For example, when preparing meat, one should monitor the temperature of the meat. If the meat is removed from the heating source and the temperature has not yet an adequate measure—the critical limit—then, the corrective action would be to return the meat to the heat source and allow it to cook until the limit was met. In some cases, such as when a food is expired, sits in the "hazard" temperature zone too long, is not frozen or reheated properly, etc., the corrective action may be to dispose of the food item.

Cleaning and sanitizing

Clean means to remove all dirt, debris, and dust from an object. For example, one may wipe a table with a cloth to remove the debris. Likewise, one may clean an object with chemical cleansing agents. Cleaning is a step in the sanitation process. An object that is sanitized, on the other hand, has been made free from microorganisms. Sanitation is achieved through employing either a chemical- or heat-based method. Therefore, items that appear to be clean may still pose a threat of illness if the objects have not been sanitized.

It is important that all kitchen equipment and utensils be thoroughly cleaned and sanitized to prevent contamination and a possible foodborne illness outbreak. Manual cleaning and sanitization of dinnerware requires a three-sink setup. Using this setup, manual cleaning and sanitization follows the following steps:
1. Scrape dinnerware to remove loose food
2. Rinse remaining food particles
3. Clean dinnerware in the first sink using warm water and detergent
4. Rinse dinnerware in second sink
5. Sanitize dinnerware in third sink using a chemical sanitizer and/or water above 175ºF. *Note: Using water that is 175ºF may pose a risk of burning to employees.
6. Air dry the dinnerware in a clean, protected area

Mechanical dish washing and sanitizing protocol includes the following steps:
1. Separate dinnerware that may not be placed in machine and/or requires special attention
2. Scrape the dinnerware free of food particles
3. Rinse dinnerware to remove remaining particles
4. Rack the dinnerware with like items only. Do not overfill the rack.
5. Wash the dinnerware by moving rack into machine and following machine directions
6. Sanitize and monitor the process, ensuring that temperature and detergent levels are adequate
7. Air dry the dishes on the rack

NSF

NSF is the acronym for National Sanitation Foundation. This foundation works to ensure food safety by granting its "seal" for equipment that is durable, cleanable, and can be fully sanitized. When purchasing food service equipment, it is wise to look for the NSF's seal, as it may guide the purchaser to products that will ultimately be safer for the organization and the consumer. Equipment that is easy to disassemble for cleaning and repair purposes is ideal. Moreover, equipment with non-absorbent, non-porous, flat services absent of crevices were food and bacteria may be trapped are preferred to those without those features. The NSF's seal may direct purchasers to these types of products.

Plumbing features

It is important that plumbing systems be properly designed and maintained in order to ensure a safe water supply for cooking and human consumptions. Certain features of a well-designed plumbing system include:
- Air-gaps. These unobstructed spaces in plumbing fixtures serve to prevent backflow. Backflow occurs when non-potable water flows into and/or mixes with potable water.
- No cross-connections. Cross-connections occur in poorly designed plumbing systems. These connections may allow contaminated water to flow and/or mix with potable water sources.
- Appropriate pressure. When a plumbing system lacks sufficient water pressure, a back-siphonage may occur. Back-siphonages are similar to backflows, however, instead of contaminated water flowing into potable water, the non-potable water is actually sucked into the potable water.

Preventing contamination of ice

Ice used during food service is easily contaminated by a variety of sources. Some methods to prevent ice contamination include:
- Store ice in a covered bin. Close cover when not in use.
- Service ice with an ice-only designated scoop. Store scoop on the outside of the ice bin (generally on the side) with handle up.
- In the event of a glass breaking in the vicinity of an ice bin, remove all ice and drain the bin. Clean thoroughly to ensure there are no shards of glass contaminating the area.

- Even when using an ice scoop, ensure hands are clean
- Clean and sanitize the ice bin, ice scoop, and any buckets used to transfer ice to the bin on a regular basis
- Use care when cleaning in the area of an ice bin. Ensure that chemicals are not sprayed in a manner that may contaminate ice.

Managing waste

As with all other aspects of food service, waste should be carefully and deliberately managed to avoid contamination of foods. Waste receptacles should be regularly cleaned, sanitized and should be fitted with tight lids. The receptacles should be free from defects which may allow leaking or seepage of discarded materials. Trash should regularly be removed from the food service area to an outdoor dumpster. Moreover, trash receptacles should be placed in the farthest possible location from food preparation areas. Outdoor dumpsters should also be fitted with tightly fitted lids, and the area surrounding the dumpsters should be maintained for cleanliness. It is also advisable to install lighting around the dumpster to ensure employee safety.

Common cleaning products

There are four primary types of cleaning supply products. The type is determined by the chemical make-up of the product. Those types are as follows:
- Alkaline detergents. These detergents are the most popularly used products and are generally used for structural services and in dishwashing machines.
- Abrasive cleaners. These cleansers are used to scour various services and may remove various types of build-up. It is important to use caution with abrasive cleansers as they may scratch services, which increases the risk of surface contamination.
- Acid products. These cleaners are most often single- or specific-use products.
- Solvent cleaners/degreasers. These products are effect at breaking down and removing grease build-up.

IPM

IPM is the acronym for integrated pest management system. Every food service organization should have an integrated pest management system in place to prevent infestation of various pests, to include (but not limited to) mice, rats, cockroaches, houseflies, ants, birds. Though these pests are small and may seem harmless, they can easily contaminate food with feces, disease, and parasites. Therefore, it is imperative that the presence of these pests be minimized and eliminated, if possible. An effective IPM does not rely on a pest control operator (also know as a pest management professional) to manage the issue of pest control, though all systems may occasionally require the services of a pest control professional.

Pest management

There are a variety of tactics that may be utilized to minimize pest infestation. Some of those tactics include:
- Maintaining clean and sanitary areas
- Store food off the floor, in airtight, pest-resistant containers
- Install screens on windows, doors, over vents, and around air ducts
- Maintain low humidity in food service areas
- Use dependable vendors who maintain an IPM for their facilities and delivery vehicles
- Install closing hinges and seals on doors and windows
- Keep a sealed lid on garbage pails
- Store food and equipment away from walls

If possible, the use of chemical agents should be avoided when attempting to manage pests in a food service setting. Chemical agents may easily contaminate food and pose a health risk for consumers. In the event that chemical solvents must be used to eradicate pests, it is important that a pest control operator who is trained and licensed in pest control management be employed. Other methods of pest eradication include using light, mechanical, and glue traps. As with all pest management systems, the most effective means of pest control is preventing access to pests, thereby preventing pest infestation.

Safety inspection checklist items

Safety inspections should be carryout at regular intervals to ensure a safe and comfortable working environment as well as to ensure product quality and safety. A safety inspection checklist may include checks regarding:
- Hot holding and hot food temperatures
- Cold holding and cold food temperatures
- Reheating, thawing, and storage temperatures
- Food preparation surface cleanliness and sanitation
- Employee safety and anti-contamination practices
- Review of labels to ensure products are labeled and dated, use of FIFO
- Chemical checklists, SDS information available

SDS

SDS (formerly MSDS) is the acronym for Safety Data Sheet. According to standards set forth by the United States Department of Labor, specifically the office of Occupational Safety and Health Administration, chemical manufacturers must produce a safety sheet for every chemical product. That safety sheet, the SDS, must be posted by employers for employee reference. SDS's must be written in English and include the following information:
- Identity (label and list, some trade secrets may be exempt)
- Chemical and common names of the product (if one ingredient)
- If multiple ingredient solvent, chemical and common names of hazardous ingredients
- Physical hazards of the material
- Medical symptoms of exposure
- Manufacturer's name and contact information

Hazard Communication Standard

The Hazard Communication Standard is a regulation enforced by the Occupational Safety and Health Administration (OSHA), an office of the U.S. Department of Labor. This standard requires employers to properly train and inform employees with regards to chemicals that may be used in the workplace. Training should include information about chemical uses and precautions, use of protective equipment, storage of chemicals, how to read an SDS (safety data sheet), and how to read product labels. If carried out properly the Hazard Communication Standard serves the organization as a whole as it may minimize the occurrence of accident, injury, and contamination by chemical means.

Daily cleaning schedule

A daily cleaning schedule is one that lists the equipment and food service areas needing daily cleaning. Each of the tasks is assigned to an employee as his/her area of responsibility for the day. Some items on the list may need to be cleaned once a day, others may need attention hourly. Utilizing a daily cleaning schedule is one method to ensure upkeep of the equipment and food service areas. By requiring employees to initial the schedule upon completion of cleaning, it also holds employees accountable for their daily duties. It is also advisable that a cleaning inspection checklist be developed in coordination with the daily cleaning schedule to ensure manager supervision over all the areas needing attention.

Utensil storage

It is important to store all clean and sanitized dinnerware in a manner that prevents contamination. Therefore, utensils stored in a cylindrical container should be placed with the handles facing upwards. Additionally, cups, bowls, and other concave dinnerware should be stored face down on clean, dry, dust-free shelves or racks. All dinnerware should be kept on clean, dry, flat, dust-free surfaces. Moreover, dinnerware should be stored off the floor and in a manner that prevents contamination from food, chemical, and other spills. Food service employees should be careful to follow proper hand washing procedure when stacking items for storage and/or accessing dinnerware to prepare a plate.

Wooden cutting boards

Wooden cutting boards are not generally recommended for food preparation, and in fact, this type of cutting board is often prohibited. Cutting boards are highly susceptible to bacteria growth and transferring foodborne pathogens as they come in contact in with a variety of foods and surfaces. For this reason, it is imperative to use cutting boards that are scratch resistant, usually of specific acrylic or rubber materials. If a cutting board shows evidence of scratching or scoring, it should immediately be replaced. Moreover, proper cleaning and sanitizing methods must be used for cutting boards to eliminate any foodborne pathogens lingering on the surface of the equipment. It is advisable to designate cutting boards for use with only one type of food, meat, vegetables, chicken, etc., to further eliminate cross-contamination.

Equipment cost analysis

An equipment cost analysis is a report comparing the cost of replacing an item to the cost of repairing said item. Repair costs should include the total costs for parts and labor. The purpose of a cost analysis is to help managers and purchasers make informed decisions regarding food service equipment. For example, if the cost of repairing an item equals or is greater to the cost of replacing an item, that item should be replaced. Additionally, careful consideration should be given to repairing items for which the repair estimates are minimally lower than the cost of replacement when the item has already had a long usage life. Cost analyses may also be used as a tool to impart the importance of performing regular preventative maintenance on all kitchen equipment.

Kitchen equipment layout

Food service areas should be designed in a manner that promotes a fast, effective flow of traffic while minimizing the need for workers to access various areas of a kitchen. Moreover, a kitchen should be laid out in such a manner that energy and light sources are effectively utilized without being overburdened. Therefore, equipment should be grouped according to function so that preparation areas are in one location, refrigerators and freezers are adjacent to one another, grills, fryers, and ovens are in convenient proximity to one another. Food preparation areas should be as far from chemical storage and cleaning areas as possible. Service areas should be designed such that food servers do not have to pass through the cooking area. Traffic areas should be wide enough to adequately handle the number of people necessary for the kitchen demand.

Equipment review

There are four nationally recognized organizations that review, approve, and certify food service equipment. Those organizations are the National Sanitation Foundation (NSF), Underwriters Laboratories (UL), American Gas Association (AGA), and International Standards Organization (ISO). NSF, UL, and AGA certify products. NSF and UL designate approval via a seal. UL approves electrical appliances. AGA grants a certification for gas appliances that meet their safety standards. Unlike the others, ISO certifies a manufacturer, not the individual products. Buying products that have met the certification standards of one or more of the above organizations ensures that a quality, inspected item is purchased.

Food service equipment safety

It is important that food service equipment be designed with safety in mind. Some equipment may have safety features built in whereas others may be fitted with extraneous parts and/or an employee may wear protective garments to ensure safety. Some standard safety equipment features include:
- Blade guards on mixers and food slicers
- Automatic shutoff for electronic equipment
- Exhaust hoods and/or other escape
- Hot service indicators
- Protective gloves, pot holders, handles, etc.
- Cord storage

Preventative maintenance program

Preventative maintenance is imperative to the longevity of food service equipment. A preventative maintenance program should be designed based upon the manufacturer's recommendations, which should be included in the appliance manual. Routine maintenance, to include cleaning and calibration, should be maintained by food service employees on a regular schedule. If necessary, a service contract should be developed for appliances requiring professional service. Records detailing all preventative maintenance should also be maintained in the event that the appliance fails while covered by a warranty. Preventative maintenance records should include appliance identifying information, such as manufacturer, model, and serial numbers, date purchased, specific appliance modifications and usage parameters, and all maintenance (to include parts and labor) performed.

Equipment safety training

Employee training is essential to a safe and productive workplace. The following items should be discussed when training employees:
- Item purpose(s)
- Protective equipment that should be worn/used during operation
- Safety concerns/procedures
- Powering on/off, basic operation, programming controls/cycles
- Special features, attachments and blades; when to use those features
- Dissembling, cleaning, sanitizing, re-assembly
- Avoiding cross-contamination
- Preventative maintenance schedule, procedures, and record keeping
- How to report equipment malfunction
- How to care for and report injuries resulting from equipment use

Manage Production

Standardized recipe

A standardized recipe is a recipe that has been tried and modified multiple times. Once the recipe meets taste and quality standards, the process is written out such that any food service employee should be able to make the recipe and produce the same results as any other food service employee. Additionally, the yield of the recipe should be equal regardless of who prepares the recipe, provided that they directly follow the written process. A standardized recipe's process should including information regarding the exact measurements of ingredients, the order that the ingredients are added to one another, and information on how to properly mix those ingredients. Additionally, a standardized recipe will include information about how to properly cook the item being served.

A standardized recipe is essential to menu planning for a variety of reasons. Some of those reasons include:
- The recipe produces a consistent yield, which ensures enough food will be made
- Every serving of the recipe will have an equal nutritional composition—regardless of when or who is prepared by
- Standardized recipes allow for more effective menu planning and food purchasing

- Food preparation time can be accurately gauged when using a standardized recipe
- A standardized recipe will result in the same product, each time it is made. Therefore, tastes, texture, and color can all be anticipated.

As a standardized recipe is used to promote consistency, it is not surprising then that every standardized recipe should contain some key elements. Those elements include:
- Name of recipe; name should be unique and descriptive
- Recipe category and number (if the organization uses a number system)
- Recipe yield
- Serving size (this is what will make the yield consistent)
- Food ingredients
- Food safety information
- Directions for mixing
- Pan size, shape, and material
- Bake time and temperature
- Serving utensils

Recipe categories

It is important that recipes be organized in a manner that is convenient and easily understood. Recipes may be organized into categories based upon the primary ingredient, so that categories may include: meats, seafood, poultry, vegetables, fruits, and others. Recipes may also be organized by the type of dish, such that categories may include: entrees, appetizers, vegetables, fruits, beverages, desserts, breads, and other categories. Or, recipes may be organized in a manner that combines the main ingredient with the type of dish, such that category offerings may include: beef entrees, poultry entrees, seafood entrees, vegetarian entrees, cake desserts, pie and pastry desserts, etc. Regardless of the method adopted by a specific organization, recipe categorization should be consistent and according to the organization's adopted policy.

Recipe scaling

Recipe scaling is integral to cooking enough food but minimizing waste. Scaling is the act of adjusting a recipe to meet the organization's needs. In some cases, scaling means cutting a recipe down and in others, it means increasing the recipe's unit of production. The below example shows how to scale a recipe (that typically yields 8 portions) to feed 214 people:
- Divide the number of servings needed by the number of servings yielded in each batch. So, $(214)/(8) = 26.75$.
- Depending upon the type of recipe, you may choose to round up to the nearest whole number. For example, one cannot easily make ¾ of a cake, so the recipe would be rounded up such that 27 batch units would be made. All ingredient amounts in the recipe would need to be multiplied by 27. Cooking/baking times might also need adjustment.

Generally speaking, it is advisable to convert measurements of ingredients from volume measurements to weight prior to scaling. This is done for multiple reasons, primary of which is ease of use. When using volume measurements, one may be dealing with multiple fractions which makes math more difficult. Moreover, measuring by weight is often quicker when making a large recipe than measuring by volume. Keep in mind that when scaling recipes, it may not be necessary to precisely scale all ingredients. Some ingredients such as butter and oil used for sautéing, spices, frostings, and others may be needed in smaller quantities than scaling might indicate.

Controlling costs with standardized recipes

The most effective way to control costs when using a standardized recipe is to follow the recipe exactly as it is written and to scale the recipe ONLY to the number of servings needed. If, for example, a cook added more meat than what was required by a recipe to avoid measuring out pre-packaged meat, the cost per serving of the meal just increased. Moreover, if an item is not properly cut into portions equaling the specified serving size, the recipe may become more costly. Larger portions result in fewer servings, which increase the cost per serving. If extra large portions are consistently served, a large portion of the kitchen budget may quickly disappear.

Proper portion sizes

Proper portioning of food results in less waste and helps to control costs. Therefore, it is important the proper portions of food are served. Proper portioning must also be done quickly to ensure temperature and taste quality of food as well as cost-effectiveness. It is advisable to use standardized food service tools such as scoops, ladles, and dishes to ensure correct portioning. Additionally, servers should cut batches into the number of servings indicated by yield, such that a pie meant to serve six is, in fact, cut into six equal pieces or a loaf of bread designed to provide 20 slices is sliced in that manner. Using correct pan sizes also ensures proper portioning.

Scoops

Listed below are the size numbers and equivalent measures of standardized scoops:
- #6 = 2/3 cup
- #8 = ½ cup
- #10 = 3/8 cup
- #12 = 1/3 cup
- #16 = ¼ cup
- #20 = 3 1/3 tablespoon
- #24 = 2 2/3 tablespoon
- #30 = 2 tablespoon
- #40 = 1 2/3 tablespoon
- #50 = 3 ¾ teaspoon
- #60 = 3 ¼ teaspoon
- #70 = 2 ¾ teaspoon
- #100 = 2 teaspoon

Forecasting

Forecasting in food services is just like weather forecasting; it is the process of predicting future needs, to include future inventory needs (and thus, purchasing needs) as well as service needs (number of portions, types of items). When forecasting, it is important to have the following types of records on-hand: previous census records, tallies, point-of-sale, and special orders/special diets. Forecasting requires knowledge of previous menus, inventories and purchases to help shape future food service needs. For example, if, in the past, portion sizes were made smaller than the suggested serving size to feed the number of people needing meals, it is helpful to have that information as direction to order additional food ingredients. Additionally, if there was access waste in the past, it may be advisable to decrease the purchase order and/or to serve a different item.

Food service sequencing

The sequence in which food is prepared, from ordering to thawing, preparing, cooking, and serving is very important for a variety of reasons. First, one must ensure that all items are on-hand and available for a planned menu. The food items must then be thawed (if necessary) such that the items are ready to be cooked but not so far in advance that the item spoils. In addition to individual food item preparatory sequencing, it is also important that a meal, as a whole follows proper sequencing, such that food items are cooked and ready for service at approximately the same time. If for example, roast beef, mashed potatoes, and salad were on a dinner menu, and all were to be served at the same time, but the roast beef was finished before the salads were prepared, the meat would cool prior to service. If, instead, the meat was prepared and left to slow cook while the salad was being prepared, the items would be finished at similar times and both would be presented at an acceptable temperature, without wilting.

Cooking terms

The following is a list of common cooking terms:
- Al dente - term used in reference to cooking pasta. It is translated from Italian to "to the tooth," and essentially means, slightly chewy.
- Bake - cooking term referring to the use of an oven for providing dry heat. Baking is most commonly used to prepare pastry goods, desserts, and casseroles.
- Baste - term used to designate that moisture should be added to foods while they cook. Typically, basting is done using pan drippings that are poured over the top of the cooking item.
- Beat - a mixing term. To beat an item means to mix it vigorously, often with a whisk or electric mixer.
- Bard - method of wrapping meat in fat before cooking
- Blackened - method of cooking food in a Cajun style, where the food is generally heavily seasoned and then cooked over high heat until charred
- Blanching - cooking method in which items are cooked using boiling water, by simmering or steaming a food or having the boiling water poured over the food
- Blend - term for combining ingredients until they reach a smooth texture and consistency
- Boil - cooking method in which a liquid is heated until it bubbles and breaks upon the surface of a liquid
- Braise - to cook food is a small amount of water or liquid while covered
- Broil - method of cooking in which food is exposed to direct, dry heat. Broiling is often done in an oven or on a grill.
- Brown - to cook food until the surface achieves a brown color. Browning may be done in some form of fat or oil and is often the first step in a longer cooking process.

- Chop - cutting term in which food is cut using a knife, food processor, or other cutting instrument into small pieces
- Clarify - method skimming a food to remove fat from the surface and/or smaller pieces from remaining fat
- Cream - mixing term in which butter or another fat is beaten until fluffy. Creaming may occur with or without an additional ingredient, such as sugar.
- Cube - cutting term in which food is cut into small, cubes
- Cut-in - method of mixing a fat with dry ingredients until small crumb-like pieces are formed
- Deglaze - method of making a sauce or gravy in which a small amount of liquid is added to a pan that meat was cooked in. As the liquid heats, the ban is scraped and the remaining food bits are combined with the liquid for flavorful sauce.
- Dicing - cutting term which refers to cutting an item into small cubes, generally smaller than the particles that result from cubing an item
- Dissolve - to mix a solid into a liquid until a homogenous solution forms and no solid remains
- Dredge - to coat a food with flour, bread crumbs, or another food. Foods are often dredged before being fried.
- Dust - cooking term for sprinkling seasoning or another dry ingredient on a food
- Fold - mixing term which means to gently blend ingredients, so as to prevent over-beating or flattening items. Folding is usually done using a light rubber spatula to sweep down and across a mixture.
- Fry - cooking method in which food is cooked in highly heated oil or fat. Deep (fat) frying is when a food is submerged in the hot oil. When little oil is used, it is called sautéing or pan frying.
- Garnish - means of dressing a plate, usually with an edible object, such as an herb, flower, chocolate or sauce. Garnish is both the act of dressing the plate as well as the term for the object dressing the plate.
- Grate - method of cutting food by rubbing it across a grater with the result being small shavings
- Grease - term for preparing a pan for cooking or baking by coating it with a layer of fat. Greasing is generally done to prevent food from sticking to the pan.
- Julienne - method of cooking in which food is cut into thin strips that are approximately the size of matches
- Knead - term for developing gluten in yeast breads. Kneading is done by folding and pressing down on dough until it results in a smooth texture.
- Macerate - term for soaking fruits or vegetables in a liquid
- Marinate - term for soaking meat in liquid in order to flavor and/or tenderize it.
- Mince - cutting term meaning to chop food into very small, irregular pieces
- Pare - term which means to peel the skin from a fruit or vegetable using a knife and/or a peeler
- Poach - cooking method in which a food is cooked in simmering water or another liquid
- Preheat - step in the cooking process in which the cook prepares the oven (or other cooking apparatus) for cooking by allowing the temperature to rise to the appropriate temperature before heating the food
- Puree - processing term meaning to cut-down, blend, or process a food until it becomes a thick liquid. The liquid is also called a puree.
- Reduce - method of thickening a sauce or liquid by allowing the water to cook off, and thus, evaporate from the fluid

- Roast - dry-heat cooking method usually applied to meats. Roasting is done without a liquid and usually completed in an oven.
- Render - term for removing fat from meat by cooking, heating, and/or straining the fat from the meat
- Sauté - cooking method in which a small amount of hot oil is used to heat and brown foods
- Score - to lightly cut the surface of a food in order to tenderize it while cooking
- Sear - cooking method in which food is quickly browned on all sides before cooking thoroughly. Searing is done to trap flavors and juices.
- Shred - cutting method in which food is taken across a shredding surface to cut small, then strips. Some foods may be shredded by hand-chopping.
- Simmer - to cook foods in liquid that is just below the boiling point
- Steam - method of cooking in which steam is used to heat food. Steaming may be done using a steaming basket, a steamer, or a pressure-cooker.
- Toss - mixing method in which foods are lightly mixed by a "tossing" or lifting and dropping motion
- Whip - mixing method in which food is mixed in a quick and light method to incorporate air into the food. Whipping is often done with a whisk, fork, mixer, or blender, and the cook should use strokes that are fast and follow an up and down pattern.
- Zest - the colorful, outer rind of citrus fruits, which is often used to add flavor to sauces, breads, pastries, and other foods. The zest is often grated to remove it from the fruit.

Food substitutions

Occasionally, it may be necessary to substitute one ingredient for another when preparing foods. This need may arise when fewer supplies than necessary were purchased, food ingredients were spoiled or contaminated, and/or delivery of food items was not timely. In the event that ingredient substitutions must be made, it is important to check the labels for similar nutritional value. Choose a substitution only if its nutritional value is comparable to the original ingredient. Remember that menus have been specially formulated to match the dietary needs of clients and failure to properly substitute may result in inadequate nutrient intake for the day.

Common food substitutions include the following:
- Baking powder, 1tsp = ½ tsp cream of tartar plus ¼ tsp baking soda
- Brown sugar (packed), 1c = 1 c granulated sugar plus 1 Tbsp molasses
- Butter = margarine; shortening
- Buttermilk, 1c = 1 Tbsp lemon juice/vinegar per 1c milk; 1c plain yogurt
- Corn syrup, 1c = 1c granulated sugar plus water
- Cornstarch, 1Tbsp (for thickening) = Flour, 1Tbsp
- Cracker crumbs = bread crumbs
- Dried beans, 1lb = 5 c cooked beans
- Granulated Sugar, 1c = 1c brown sugar; 2c powdered sugar
- Milk, 1c = ¼-1/3c dry milk plus 1c water; ½c evaporated milk plus 1c water

*Note: Substitutions may effect quality or taste of finished product.

Testing and evaluating new recipes

Testing recipes, often several times, prior to service is important to ensure that the recipe is properly prepared, is time and cost effective, and meets the quality expectations of an organization. Testing a recipe is also an important part of recipe modification and standardization. During test runs, a recipe should be tried by a panel of individuals, who then evaluate the food on taste, texture, appearance, and recommendations for modification. If the food is not appealing, the recipe may be modified or the recipe rejected. A recipe may be further tested upon service to clients. Ask customers to evaluate new foods by responding to a survey. After reviewing all of the survey results, decide whether a recipe should remain on a menu, be modified or discarded.

Edible yield

Edible yield is the percentage of a product that remains available for production and edible after the initial preparation takes place. For example, if an apple filling were to be made from whole apples, the edible yield would be the percentage that remained after paring and coring the apple. The remaining fruit would also comprise the net weight of the edible parts. Therefore, edible yield may be affected by how an ingredient is packaged and will be used. Canned goods, for example, will have a lower drain weight (weight of portion remaining after liquid/syrup is drained) than they do package weight. Fruits and vegetables that must be cored and/or pared will have a smaller net weight after being prepped. The edible yield of meats may be affected by the amount of fat on a portion. When factoring purchase needs, it is important that the edible yield factor be taken into consideration.

Minimum/maximum inventory system

A minimum/maximum inventory system operates such that certain items are always kept on-shelf and that the minimum and/or maximum amount on-hand always falls within a pre-determined range. This system works well in that it ensures a sufficient supply of staples are on hand. That being said, it is slightly more complicated than one may initially believe as the person performing and inventory must take into account the number of item units that will be used prior to receiving the next shipment of goods. Additionally, one must factor lead time on ordered products as well as the rate at which current will get used. A minimum/maximum inventory should only be used for non-perishable items, as even when following "first in, first out" principles, certain items may sit for an extended period of time.

Par level inventory system

The par level inventory system and the minimum/maximum inventory system are similar in that both specify a minimum desired inventory requirement. However, a par level system does not have a maximum per unit requirement. So, in many senses, a par level inventory is a much simpler inventory, as one may take stock of the current inventory and order enjoy supplies to bring the inventory back up to "par," or the minimum desired per unit inventory. This system does not require as much calculation, as lead units does not necessarily affect the purchase order. A par level inventory, however, is not as flexible as a minimum/maximum inventory, and therefore, should only be used with established menus and forecasts.

Perpetual inventory system

A perpetual inventory system is a method of inventory accounting that operates much like a checking account ledger, in that a perpetual inventory depends heavily on record keeping and equalizing purchases and withdrawals. A perpetual inventory system works such that as an item unit is used, a new unit of equal quantity is ordered. Before initiating a perpetual inventory system, a thorough inventory is of stock is performed. The number of units of each item is the existing balance of said item. When an item is used, the number of units used are subtracted from the balance. When an item is received, the number of items received are added to the balance. Once the inventory is established, it may be effective to simply total the number of units withdrawn from the previous menu cycle and reorder that same number of units for the future. It is important, however, that spot inventories continue to take place to ensure accurate and honest accounting of inventory stock.

Calculating lead units

Lead units are the number of units of an item that are ordered in anticipation of inventory being used. So, to calculate lead units, one must first calculate lead time and usage rates and compare those numbers to the minimum/maximum inventory range. Lead time refers to the time that passes between ordering a product and receiving that item. So, if three days pass between the date on which cases of beans were ordered and when they were received, then the lead time is three days. Usage rate may be calculated by estimating the number of units that will be used over a given period of time. So, in this case, we'll say that one case of beans is used every three days. Which means, during the lead time (three days), one case will be used. So, to maintain current inventory, at least one lead case (unit) should be added to the purchase order.

Shrinkage and other discrepancies

It is not uncommon to have inventory shrink contrary to that indicated by the number of units actually used to prepare menus. Some circumstances that may lead to inventory discrepancies include:
- Inventory items are lost or misplaced by the shipment receiver. This may occur if the employee is not familiar with the kitchen layout and/or when an item is hidden by other items in the area.
- Inventory items are stolen by anyone having access to the kitchen
- Food items are spoiled or contaminated. This may occur when food is not properly rotated, is improperly stored, the package is damaged, is not consumed in a timely manner, and/or contamination occurs during food service.
- Error occurred during initial inventory
- Employee receiving food did not verify purchase orders against received shipment

Determining equipment needs

Before investing in new equipment for the kitchen, it is first important to consider a variety of criteria to ensure that the final purchase is a wise one. Some pre-purchase equipment consideration criteria include the following:
- Specific needs; equipment use(s)
- Existing equipment function/compatibility

- Available space, power sources
- Ease of use, cleaning, sanitation
- Durability of materials
- Price, warranty, support services provided
- Safety features to avoid employee injury
- Design/features that reduce risk of food contamination
- Available budget
- Additional features/functions
- Other equipment that must be purchased in order to maintain or operate

Manage Business Operations

Purchase specification

Purchase specifications define the parameters in which various characteristics of a food or product should fall such that purchase of that item is wise, acceptable, and beneficial to an organization. These specifications are developed in order to ensure safe and quality purchases are made. Purchase specification factors for meat, poultry, and fish may include the following characteristics:
- Type of item (fish, poultry)
- Inspection
- Grade
- Style, form
- Refrigeration state/requirements
- Processing needs
- Weight
- Age
- Quality, to include: Fat, Color, Eyes, Skin, Gills

Before buying any food, it is important to compare the vendor's product to the purchase specifications set forth by the organization for which the food is being purchased. Checking purchase specifications ensures that purchases meet a quality standard that is acceptable to the organization. Shop vendors until products are found that meet all of the purchase specifications. Compromising these specifications may compromise the safety and quality of a food. Purchase specifications for fresh and processed produce include the following characteristics:
- Grade
- Size
- Type
- Drain weight (if applicable)
- Quantity
- Packaging unit
- Packaging material/methods
- Growing region

Food purchases must take into account the gross product after drain weight, coring, paring, de-boning cooking, and other procedures occur, as that product is likely to be significantly less than the as purchased weight. As purchase weight accounts for the net weight of a product, while in packaging. This weight includes peels, skins, cores, juices/syrups, water, bones, fat, etc. Once those additional materials are discarded and/or separated, the edible portion of a food remains. Edible portions may also be affected during cooking as most foods "cook down." In order to properly estimate inventory needs, one must first calculate the edible yield factor, which is equivalent to the product once the weight of the edible portion is divided by the as purchased weight. The edible yield factor may then be used to better approximate food costs and purchasing needs.

Product specification

Product specifications should include information that may be useful in choosing vendors and their products. The specifications act as guidelines, and as such, they should outline the desirable characteristics of a product, such as color, grading, weight, composition, and other information. Specifications need to be clear and specific but not so restrictive that it becomes impossible to find "quality" products. Specifications are used not only to select food but also as a tool for the vendor to cater products and prices to the needs of an organization. Specifications should include information including the name of the product, its primary uses, its characteristics, the quality of the product, procedures for receiving the product and a section for special notes and consideration, such as storage, preparation, quality, etc.

Purchase order information

Purchase orders are necessary for the requisition of goods and services. Purchases orders commonly have the following information:
- Supplier information to include name, address, phone and fax numbers
- Shipping/delivery point of contact, location
- Order number
- Order date
- Delivery date
- Item name
- Item description
- Unit type
- Number of units
- Cost per unit
- Total cost per item
- Subtotal of order
- Taxes (if applicable)
- Shipping/delivery charges
- Total cost of order
- Payment information

Competitive bidding

Competitive bidding is a process by which an organization may choose a vendor(s) for certain products and services. The process relies heavily on preparation by the organization that is receiving bids, in that to provide an organization with the most complete and accurate bids, the organization must first determine product specifications for a vendor to meet. The vendor then prepares a price quote for the products and services that it is asked to provide. It is important to remember that the quote is based on the specifications, to include quantity and quality, of items and changes in these specifications may affect the quoted bid. If carried out effectively, competitive bidding will often result in the selection of a high quality, lower cost vendor.

Computer use

Computer use is mainstream, and if used correctly, computers may be a helpful tool to any organization. Computers aid in streamlining processes, communication, file sharing, document preparation, file storage, and many other applications. Currently, there are many software applications available which are designed specifically for food service operations, though generic word processing, spreadsheet, and database programs may suit the organization's needs. Once software is learned and document processes implemented, a computer may eliminate costs by reducing man-hours required by purchasing and inventory applications, scheduling, forecasting, menu planning, and so many other tasks. Specifically designed, food service/dietary management, computer software is available. The features, cost, and ease of use vary from program to program, so it is important that several programs be researched prior to purchase.

Common features dietary management software include:
- Meal service features, including ticket/tray-line preparation, payment systems, allergies and drug interactions, etc.
- Menu planning features, including menu-cycle features, creating a visually appealing menu chart, balancing a menu, etc.
- Forecasting features, including automatic forecasting, food-waste analysis
- Purchasing features, including easy purchase orders, cost tracking, etc.
- Inventory applications, including management processes, monitoring, etc
- Food production applications, food prep timelines, rotations, scheduling, etc.
- Financial resources, including payroll, cost analyses, etc
- Safety features, including mandatory reporting information and forms, contamination information, and resources regarding food safety

Regardless of the documentation methods employed by a specific organization, it is imperative that all confidential information be protected against unauthorized access, which may include access by employees, visitors, hackers, and other computer users. This concern becomes paramount when utilizing the internet, even for "web-surfing" purposes. Therefore, it is important to ask software vendors for information regarding file protection, to include software controls such as password protected logins. Additionally, work with the internet provider to ensure that the organizations has a secure internet connection and that firewalls and other security features are in place. Moreover, information that is stored on a computer and/or any other type of media should not only be protected by password but also by storing the data management system in a safe, locked location.

Cash bank system

When working with cash, it is important to implement systems and procedures that ensure employee honesty and accountability. One such method is using a new cash bank for each cashier and/or money handler. When a cashier clocks in for his/her shift, the cashier is then given a new "bank" with a predetermined amount of money in the "bank." He or she then counts the cash and signs for the drawer. At the end of the shift, the cashier and his/her supervisor recount the cash in the drawer and reconcile it against the original bank amount plus the total amount of transactions. The money in the drawer should equal the sum of the bank and transactions. Discrepancies must be clearly documented. Both the cashier and his/her supervisor sign off on the turned in bank. If the amount of cash in the drawer is consistently less than that indicated by the transaction record the employee may need additional training on keying entries and/or may be pocketing money.

Security procedures for handling cash

It is important to implement various financial security procedures to protect against theft. Unfortunately, employees, including managers and supervisors, clients, and guests are all capable of committing theft. However, implementation of security procedures such as those listed below may deter such crime:
- Keep excess cash in a safe. Allow access to as few individuals as possible (though there should be at least two, for accountability purposes).
- Use locking cash drawers. Keep drawers closed when not performing transactions.
- Give each cashier his/her own bank at the start of a shift
- Minimize the amount of money allowed in registers at any given time
- Limit the amount of money employees may carry on their person
- If employees may be exiting the facility with large sums of cash, ensure adequate lighting and recommend the "buddy system"

Minimizing costs and theft

In most cases, organizations can minimize product and monetary theft by implementing a checks-and-balances or buddy system. Such systems eliminate the possibility that one individual is ordering, receiving, and inventorying items, which makes it easy for that individual to walk away with goods. After foods are purchased, it is advisable to have another employee receiving the items. This individual should verify the product units as well as the quantity of units against the purchase order. If the order is received as specified in the order, he or she should sign off on said order. Otherwise, the purchaser and/or a supervisor need to be contacted. Likewise, when performing an inventory, a team comprised of at least two employees should be surveying, documenting, and singing off on inventory items. Inventory discrepancies should then be resolved by a third party. Additionally, inventory spot-checks and use of security cameras are all wise security measures.

Revenue-generating services

Revenue-generating services are any services which produce income or profit for an organization. Depending upon the type of organization, the revenue may be realized purely as profit or may be a means to expand service offerings. Because many institutions provide meals as part of the overall service provided, revenue generating services are often more creative. Some examples of institutional revenue-generating services include:

- Snack and/or coffee carts
- Snack, soda, and other vending machines
- Specials treats, such as popcorn and sodas during movies
- Catering options
- Meals/snacks available to visitors
- Meals/snacks available to employees
- Special occasion meal and/or banquet

As the name suggests, revenue-generating services are only affective if income is realized. Therefore it is important to manage the services in such a way as to maximize profit and minimize expense. Expenses that may be incurred during the implementation of revenue-generating services may include the following:

- Marketing and advertising, to include fliers, newsletters, signs, commercials, product promotion, taste-tests, and other
- Additional labor costs, to include everything from recipe development to production to packaging
- Packaging and utensil costs (especially for take-out and specialty items)
- Equipment and service costs
- Decoration, linen, and dinnerware costs for catered events

For revenue-generating services to be effective, others must know about them. This requires internal and external marketing and advertising. Some advertising methods that may be effective include: print media, such as posters, banners, fliers, and signs, in and outside of the organization; promotions, to include taste-tests, open houses, raffles/drawings/contests, discounts; fairs targeting the appropriate audiences; radio and television commercials; web-based advertising. The most effective marketing of any service is done through word-of-mouth, as it is based upon recommendations from previous customers. Offer customers future discounts for referrals. Ask for letters of reference from satisfied customers and add these to the marketing portfolio. Additionally, if revenue will be used towards new programming and/or philanthropic goals, be sure to mention this is advertising. Customers often prefer giving business to a worthy cause vice someone's pockets.

In order to effectively price a food item, one must first calculate the food cost. This is done by adding the raw food cost plus labor plus other miscellaneous expenses. Take that sum and divide it by the serving yield for a per serving food cost. After the food cost is determined, a mark-up, generally between 30-65% is added to the cost. This is done by multiplying the food cost by (100% + mark-up). If the product is an odd figure and/or does not match the organization's pricing convention, it should be adjusted accordingly. When pricing an item for revenue-generating services, it is important to also perform a market analysis which lists the price for comparable items at local restaurants and institutions. A market analysis will ensure that food items are priced within a reasonable profit margin.

Pricing may also be influenced by the goal of the organization. If the revenue from the food is meant to subsidize a program it may be priced differently than if the food is being used purely as a means of generating profit revenues.

Catering events

Catering events can seriously boost revenue if done in a cost-effective manner. Typically speaking, costs of catered events will include:
- Food costs
- Labor costs, covers costs per hour per laborer
- Location, equipment, service linens and dinnerware rental and/or purchase fees

To make a catered event cost-effective, the food costs must first be determined by multiplying the costs per serving by the number of individuals on the projected guest lists. Next, labor costs, to include food preparation, service, and facility preparation and clean up, must be added to the total of food costs. Finally, facility and equipment rental fees round out the sum. To generate revenue, then, that sum must be marked up by a pre-determined percentage. Thus, to generate 20% revenue, one would multiply the sum of the costs by 1.2. The product would be the cost quote for the event.

Clients may ask for a price-per-serving estimate for catered events in order to better compare the services of one organization to that of another. Price per serving is determined by calculating the sum of the event costs, multiplying that number by the revenue markup and dividing the product by the number of servings. See the simplified example below to figure the cost per serving for an event with the following figures:
- Raw food costs = $9.72/person
- Labor costs = $78.00/hour
- Room rental fee = $50.00/hour
- Revenue markup 45%
- Number of guests = 55
- Number of labor hours = 5
- Number of rental hours = 3
- Cost of event = ($9.72 x 55) + ($78.00 x 5) + ($50.00 x 3) =$1074.60
- Price of event = $1072.60 x 1.45 = $1558.17
- Price-per-serving = $1558.17 / 55 = $28.33

*Note: Some organizations may choose to figure the price-per-serving without including the rental fee and then adding that fee as an additional expense.

Catering event menus may be pre-determined by the organization or truly specific to the event. While a pre-set menu may be beneficial to the institution, as it limits food costs, it may feel too structured to some clients. Therefore, it is wise to give the client at least a selective menu to choose from. Selective menus may limit the options to certain, often prepared items to make the event more cost- and time-effective while still seeming very flexible, as the client is able to "mix-and-match" to suit their organizations needs. It may also be helpful to develop "themed" menus. Doing so will allow for specific types of meals, with tried and true recipes as well as an eclectic and collection of colored linens and decoration. Having barbeque, holiday, springtime brunch (think Mother's Day, Easter, etc), and other themes on-hand and ready to go may pay for both the institution and the client.

Capital equipment

Capital equipment is equipment that has a significant purchase price (different organizations define the price differently—some say $500, some more or less) and a long-life expectancy. Capital equipment is often essential to the organization and/or significantly cuts the labor costs of an organization, thus justifying the higher sticker price. In addition to reducing labor costs, capital equipment purchases are often justified by comparing the costs of maintenance and repair of older equipment to the purchase price and warranty of new equipment. Additionally, many newer appliances significantly cut energy costs, which, in the long term, could make purchase of a newer model worthwhile.

When shopping for capital equipment replacement, it is important to compare brands, models, features, and prices of available equipment. Cheaper brands or models may not carry the warranty or features of more expensive brands. Likewise, some equipment may be backed by service support. Before purchasing any capital equipment, it is wise to do market research, ask for recommendations, and perform side-by-side comparisons of the equipment. This research will help one formulate a budget justification for capital equipment as the individual will be familiar with the features that justify the purchase. Budget justifications should include information about warranties, service support, cost- and time-savings, savings over repairing older equipment, and information about the safety features of the capital equipment. If the budget justification is approached as a document that proves the long term savings generated by capital equipment, the purchase is more likely to be approved.

Capital equipment may come in all shapes and sizes and be for all purposes. Depending upon the price minimum that an organization puts on capital equipment, some examples of such equipment include:
- Refrigerators
- Freezers
- Mixers
- Cutters
- Slicers
- Steam tables
- Steam kettles
- Food transport and delivery systems
- Beverage dispensers
- Ovens
- Fryers
- Griddles
- Cutlery sets
- Pot sets
- Food processors
- Butcher tables/stations
- Preparation stations
- Specialty items
- Bread makers
- Warmers

Evaluating vendor performance

It is important to work with reliable and reputable vendors, as their ability and willingness to provide the organization with necessary products and services affects the organization's ability to provide quality customer service as well. Vendors should be evaluated on a variety of criteria, to include:

- Ability to acquire necessary and desired products in a timely manner and at quoted costs
- Makes scheduled deliveries, works with organization to schedule convenient deliveries
- Follow-through on orders, promised goods
- Provides quality customer service
- Upholds any contracts, service agreements, and understandings/obligations
- Works with the organization to ensure safety for employees and customers
- Provides high quality products at a competitive price

Purchasing and receiving

In order to ensure employee honesty and accountability, a person not responsible for food purchases should receive food and other products. This individual should check the purchase order against the delivered items and delivery invoice. Any discrepancies should be brought to the attention of the vendor as well as the purchaser for rectification. After all purchased items are accounted for in the delivery, the receiver will sign off on the delivery invoice. It is important to separate the purchasing and receiving duties in order to avoid employee theft and/or embezzlement. Additionally, it is important that inventory also be done by a separate party from the purchaser and receiver. Again, this practice is advisable in that it promotes employee accountability and ensures fewer product accounting errors are made.

Budget

A budget is essential a financial plan that outlines the expenditure allowances and revenue estimates. Expenditures, or expenses, are the monies that are paid out to vendors, employees, and for other costs. Revenues are the monies coming in. Budgets should, at minimum, break even, such that the revenues at least meet the expenses. It is desirable and smart to minimize expenses and maximize revenues such that revenues exceed expenses and a profit is generated. This profit may go back into providing additional and/or enhanced goods or services or it may be distributed among company share holders. In food service, the most significant expenses often include food and labor costs. Additional expenses may include supplies, capital equipment, maintenance, and utility costs. Revenue may be generated by a variety of services which may include anything from catering to vending services.

To revise a budget, it is important to first review records of previous budgets, analyzing the success of those budgets. Also, do a review of market trends to determine whether food costs have increased or decreased and by how much. Estimate what the department needs will be for the coming year, to include additional labor costs, replacing and/or maintaining capital equipment, as well as utility, rental, and other fees. Determine whether the organization will continue with the same vendor(s) or a new vendor(s). Initiate a new bidding process. Consider the season and any factors that may have influenced crop and/or product yields. Determine new services that will be offered and the costs of those services. Then, using the previous budget as a starting point, determine which budget expenses will likely increase, decrease or stay the same. Add or subtract the percentage increase or decrease that research and experience dictates for each budget item (be sure to work with a specific, categorized budget). It is advisable to add a bit of padding to a budget, without overshooting too greatly to ensure financial needs are met through the coming budget period.

Food cost

It is easiest and often most effective to calculate food cost for a period of time. In this instance, let's use a menu cycle of six weeks. To calculate food costs over a period of time, it is important to have a well reconciled inventory. Using that documentation, take the inventory value at the start of the period. For this example, beginning inventory was $10,000. Add to that figure the inventory growth or purchases over the period (in this case six weeks). Inventory growth was $9,000. Subtract the ending inventory value. End value, for this example, was $11,000. So for this example, the food cost of a six week cycle was $10,000 + $9,000 - $11,000 = $8,000 in food costs.

To determine percentage of food costs, divide the total amount of food costs by the total amount allocated for food or generated by food revenue. So, for this cycle, if $23,000 was allocated for food services, then food costs equaled 34%. (Calculation: ($8,000 / $23,000) x 100 = 34%)

As with other areas in food service, savings to the organization means greater revenue generated. Food cost savings may be generated by:
- Using standardized recipes, properly scaled
- Avoid preparing, purchasing, or serving excess food
- Prices of prepared foods versus those that must be prepare in-house
- Monitor employees to ensure food is not stolen or eaten
- Save, store, and serve leftovers, if possible
- Monitor plate waste, conduct taste-testing panels
- Analyze and compare recipe costs, vendor bids
- Choose menu items that are in-season
- Reduce food spoilage and contamination - Employ safety practices, use "first in, first out" practices, monitor temperatures during delivery and service

Daily cost per meal

In some cases, a manager may be given a budget per individual to be served. This may be one instance in which the manager would need to determine the cost per meal. Determining costs per meal is similar to other costs calculations in that first the raw food and preparation costs for prepared meals must be determined. Then, the manager will use the census, or the total number of customers served, to determine the cost per meal. The raw costs are divided by the census. This gives a cost per meal. Likewise, a cost per client per day can be figured by adding the costs per meals served throughout the day. Each organization has different needs, and therefore, each organization may require various calculations as part of budget justification, pricing, and for other reasons. It is important that a dietary manager be able to break down basic calculations and/or utilize computer software to provide data to finance departments.

Departmental cost-saving practices

Departments can minimize and control costs in a variety of ways. Some of those ways include the following:

- Carefully schedule employees to ensure adequate but not overly-abundant coverage of necessary areas
- Avoid scheduling employees overtime
- Train employees in order to streamline processes, prevent errors and overuse of various products
- Provide service only during select hours of the day
- Reduce labor costs by purchasing prepared foods, capital equipment, etc.
- Utilize computer systems to generate reports, orders, and monetary inventories
- Encourage employees to use products sparingly, if able
- Offer employee incentives based upon revenues generated
- Develop and utilize energy-saving procedures - Turn off lights and appliances when not in use, maintain insulation around doors and openings of heating and refrigerating units, insulate windows and doors of kitchen

Monetary rewards

Employees are motivated by room for growth, salary increase, and other incentives. It is important that an organization encourage employees in this manner. Organizations can do that by establishing job descriptions and goals for employees. These descriptions and goals should be discussed and evaluated during performance reviews. Employees should be given direction as to how they may improve their performance and should be given the opportunity to learn about the skills and achievements needed in order to attain a promotion. Raises and bonuses should be awarded based upon employee performance, merit, education, and any other criteria set forth by an organization.

Practice Test

Practice Questions

1. A resident is admitted to a long-term care facility. The initial nutrition assessment is completed on day 8 and is charted in the progress note section of the medical record. A week later, an error is noticed in the nutrition assessment, involving the height and weight of the resident. Correction fluid (White Out) is used to correct the error, and a follow-up note is placed in the chart. What is wrong in this situation?
   a. The nutrition assessment should be placed in the dietary section
   b. The nutrition assessment should be documented on day 14
   c. Correction fluid (White Out) should never be used in a medical record
   d. The accuracy of height and weight is not important

2. A diet history is needed for a client who is admitted to a nursing home. Generally accepted methods for obtaining this information include all of the following EXCEPT a:
   a. 24-hour recall
   b. 7-day food diary
   c. Food frequency questionnaire
   d. 3-day food record

3. The main purpose of nutrition screening is to identify individuals who may:
   a. Be at risk for malnutrition
   b. Need to lose weight
   c. Not be getting enough calcium
   d. Not be drinking enough fluids

4. Which of the following laboratory values indicates dehydration?
   a. Serum sodium of 155 mEq/L
   b. Serum sodium of 130 mEq/L
   c. Serum albumin of 3.6 g/dL
   d. Serum potassium of 4 mEq/L

5. The physician has ordered a low-fiber diet for a resident who is experiencing a flare-up of diverticulitis. How would the following breakfast menu be modified to meet the changes ordered by the physician?
   - ½ cup all-bran cereal
   - 1 toasted English muffin
   - 1 banana
   - ½ cup orange juice
   - ½ cup low-fat milk
   - 1 cup of coffee
   a. Eliminate the orange juice
   b. Eliminate the English muffin
   c. Change the banana to prunes
   d. Change the cereal to corn flakes

6. A resident who is Muslim is admitted to a health care facility. The physician orders a diet consisting of mechanical soft, high protein and no concentrated sweets. Which of the following lunch menus is most appropriate for this resident?

    a. Tuna sandwich, tapioca pudding, and apple juice

    b. Hotdog, potato chips, fresh fruit cup, and low-fat milk

    c. Meatloaf made from ground beef, mashed potatoes, steamed carrots, unsweetened canned pears, and low-fat milk

    d. Spaghetti and meatballs, salad with ranch dressing, bread, butter, and ginger ale

Questions 7 & 8 pertain to the following passage:

    Mary has been a resident at a long-term care facility for 3 months. She is on a regular diet, has no acute nutritional issues, is able to feed herself, and is maintaining her admission weight.

7. When does Mary require her nutritional care plan to be reviewed and updated?

    a. Every month

    b. Quarterly

    c. Every week

    d. Every 6 months

8. The dietary manager has completed the review of Mary's care plan. Two weeks later, Mary refuses meals complaining of having no appetite. The nursing staff reports that she is losing weight. The dietary manager should next do which of the following?

    a. Wait until the next quarterly evaluation to intervene

    b. Ask the nurses to let the dietary manager know if the situation does not improve within 2 weeks

    c. Immediately update Mary's nutrition care plan with an intervention to address her lack of appetite and weight loss

    d. Ask the physician for an order for nutritional supplements to be sent to the resident twice a day

9. In an assisted living facility with 75 beds, the dietary manager is most likely to choose which of the following menus for a varied population with many different diet restrictions?

    a. Nonselective menu

    b. Selective menu

    c. Semiselective menu

    d. Static menu

10. A patient's wife has requested information from the dietary manager, regarding a heart healthy diet to lower cholesterol for her own information. What would be the most appropriate materials to provide to the patient?

    a. Find any web site on the Internet that has information that can be printed

    b. Tell the woman her request cannot be accommodated without an order from her physician

    c. Provide the woman with information on reducing sodium in her diet

    d. Provide some simple materials that concern fat in the diet from the American Heart Association and the name of a dietitian

11. A 70-year-old patient has been admitted for short-term rehab as a result of a fractured hip. He has a history of type 2 diabetes that is controlled with medication. After interviewing this patient, it appears that he has not been following any special diet because he feels that the medication should be taking care of the blood sugar. The dietary manager is asked to begin to educate him on the appropriate diet. What are ways in which to evaluate the progress of this patient while he is a patient in the rehab facility?
    a. Ask the patient yes and no questions every week to see if he can answer correctly
    b. Provide the patient with a regular selective menu, and review his menu choices daily, making corrections as needed to meet his dietary requirements
    c. Provide the patient with a follow-up quiz that he can complete at his leisure since he will be staying for a few weeks
    d. Set goals for the patient, and then check with him the week that he is scheduled for discharge to assess progress

12. Many of the residents of a nursing home require minced or pureed meals because they have chewing and swallowing issues. What factors should be taken into account when planning meals?
    a. The USDA's MyPlate should be followed as closely as possible with care taken to present the food as attractively as possible
    b. The standard menu selections should be put in the blender and pureed and then served to residents with a diet order of puree/minced
    c. All foods can be prepurchased as baby food, according to the specific texture ordered
    d. The food items on the regular diet can be pureed and served as most of these residents will not know the difference anyway due to dementia or inability to communicate effectively

13. Oral nutritional supplements are appropriate in a patient who is:
    a. Having difficulty swallowing
    b. Experiencing a 6% weight loss
    c. Requesting "milkshakes"
    d. On a "no concentrated sweets" diet

14. A number of complaints have been received about the meals in a health care facility. Options for continuous quality improvement to address this issue include all of the following EXCEPT:
    a. Plate waste studies
    b. Patient surveys
    c. Test trays
    d. Employee surveys

15. All of the following is information that may be obtained in a patient satisfaction survey EXCEPT:
    a. Opinions on the temperature of the food and timing of meals
    b. Perceptions on the service received from the food service employees
    c. Opinions on the cost of meals and suggestions for improvements
    d. Opinions on the menu selections and tray accuracy

16. The standard serving size for mashed potatoes is one-half cup. The scoop used to serve this portion is a:
   a. #6 scoop
   b. #8 scoop
   c. #12 scoop
   d. #16 scoop

17. Consider the following scheduling parameters: three employees work 8-hour shifts 5 days a week, ten employees work 5-hour shifts 4 days a week, six employees work 8-hour shifts 3 days a week, and one employee works on weekends only with 8-hour shifts. This schedule accounts for how many full time equivalents (FTEs)?
   a. 10 FTEs
   b. 12 FTEs
   c. 15 FTEs
   d. 20 FTEs

18. The document that lists the job responsibilities and duties as well as the skills required for a particular position is called a job:
   a. Specification
   b. Analysis
   c. Description
   d. Title

19. When interviewing an applicant for a cashier position which requires long hours standing, which of the following interview questions would be considered inappropriate or illegal?
   a. Was there even a situation in your last job where you had to handle an angry customer?
   b. Why did you leave your last job?
   c. How do you feel about the fact that this position requires standing in one place for long periods of time?
   d. What a beautiful engagement ring. Are you getting married soon?

20. The tray-line checker in the kitchen is not performing her job effectively. There are many missing items from the tray that are not caught by this employee. Initial steps this employee's supervisor may take to address this issue include all of the following EXCEPT a:
   a. Performance improvement plan
   b. Corrective action
   c. Letter of termination
   d. Review of her job description

21. The name of the law that helps to protect workers and job applicants who are age 40 and older from discrimination based on their age is called the:
   a. Age Discrimination in Employment Act of 1967
   b. Civil Rights Act of 1964
   c. Older Americans and Gender Discrimination Act of 1963
   d. Equal Pay Act of 1963

22. Which of the following scenarios would be in violation of the Food and Drug Administration Food Code of 2009?
   a. The food service employee has used a printed a label on the computer, indicating that the bulk container holds corn flakes and that the product was manufactured in a plant that also processes peanut-containing products
   b. An employee had a plethora of zucchini during the summer and decided to bake zucchini bread at home. The supervisor on duty thought it would be a good addition to the breakfast offerings for residents
   c. The head cook used a clean spoon to taste the gravy he has prepared then places the utensil in the dirty equipment area
   d. At a residential home for adolescents, steak is a weekly menu choice cooked to an internal temperature of 150°F

23. The dietary manager of a small kitchen at a convalescent home must revise the menu and asks all employees to join a staff meeting to discuss their ideas and suggestions. After considering all input, the dietary manager selects a few new menu items to begin recipe development. This style of management is called:
   a. Authoritative managing
   b. Proactive managing
   c. Participative managing
   d. Autocratic managing

24. A food service supervisor at a rehabilitation hospital overhears a tray-line employee discussing a high-profile athlete who has been admitted for rehab following an automobile accident. This is a violation of which of the following federal laws?
   a. Federal Privacy Act of 1997
   b. Family Educational Rights and Privacy Act
   c. Consumer and Patient Right to Privacy Act
   d. Health Insurance Portability and Accountability Act of 1996

25. Which of the following situations will likely cause a citation from the state health inspector?
   a. Chicken thawing in the refrigerator
   b. Food in the warming trays held at a temperature of 140°F
   c. Raw meat in the walk-in refrigerator stored on the shelf above the fresh produce
   d. The temperature in the walk-in refrigerator between 38°F and 40°F

26. A dietary manager of a long-term care facility who frequently visits with the residents during meals notices that one man seems to be drooling and coughing while eating. Which of the following referrals may be required?
   a. Occupational therapy
   b. Physical therapy
   c. Recreational therapy
   d. Speech therapy

27. The consulting dietitian is attending a care planning session. She learns that residents on one wing of the nursing home are served breakfast at 9 a.m., lunch at 12:30 p.m., and dinner at 5 p.m. Evening snacks are not routinely offered because residents in the past have refused any snack other than a cup of hot tea. The dietitian has alerted the director of food services that this may be in violation of federal regulations. What is the best way to address this issue?

    a. Add a nourishing evening snack at 8 p.m.
    b. Move the dinner meal to 6 p.m.
    c. Move the breakfast meal to 8 a.m.
    d. Move the lunch meal to 1 p.m.

28. To meet federal regulations, which require a dietitian for a nursing home, appropriate choices include all of the following EXCEPT a:

    a. Full-time registered dietitian
    b. Food service director
    c. Registered dietitian employed on a consultant basis
    d. Registered, licensed dietitian employed part-time

29. Which of the following United States Department of Agriculture grades are used for poultry?

    a. US Prime, Choice, Select, or Standard
    b. US Grades A, B, or C
    c. US Fancy, Extra No. 1, No. 1, No. 2, or Combination
    d. US Fancy, Choice, Standard, or Substandard

30. Which of the following cooking methods is preferable for Select grade beef?

    a. Frying
    b. Grilling
    c. Oven roasting
    d. Braising

31. A dietary manager conducting an inspection of the dry storage area should be most concerned about:

    a. Canned goods that are stored on metal shelving
    b. Large bags of rice that are stored on the floor
    c. Open bags of flour and sugar that are stored in covered containers
    d. The food that has just been delivered is placed at the back of the shelves

32. A dietary manager who is doing inventory in the walk-in refrigerator finds that the temperature log indicates a range of 36°F–38°F. Which of the following food items would need to be discarded?

    a. Ground beef that is 2 days old
    b. Fresh eggs that are 2 weeks old
    c. Poultry that is 5 days old
    d. Fresh fish that is 1 day old

33. All of the following statements about *Escherichia coli* infection are true EXCEPT:
    a. It can be spread through contaminated food and water
    b. It is one of the most common food-borne illnesses
    c. It most often presents with nausea and vomiting
    d. It can be spread through contaminated swimming pools

34. Where is the most appropriate initial place to report an outbreak of a *Salmonella* infection?
    a. Local health department
    b. Centers for Disease Control
    c. Food and Drug Administration
    d. The local health clinic

35. Which of the following foods are least likely to cause food-borne illness?
    a. Raw eggs
    b. Medium rare roast beef
    c. Raw shellfish
    d. Fresh fruits and vegetables

36. As part of the yearly retraining for food service staff on preventing food-borne illness, which of the following points are appropriate to include in the training?
    a. When preparing food, it is important to use a different knife and cutting board when chopping vegetables and raw meat
    b. Produce can be served as is because it is washed at the facility from where it is shipped
    c. Frequent hand washing is one of the best defenses against food-borne illness
    d. A and C above

37. For what does the acronym OSHA stand?
    a. Occupational Safety and Hazard Administration
    b. Occupational Safety and Health Administration
    c. Office of Sanitation and Health Accounts
    d. Office of Safety and Health Administration

38. After doing a thorough inspection of the dish machine, including the temperature, detergents, and the wash cycle, which of the following measurements would be a cause for concern?
    a. Wash temperature of 180°F
    b. Hot water sanitizing rinse temperature of 180°F
    c. Chemical sanitizing (chlorine) final rinse temperature of 117°F
    d. Hot water sanitizing final rinse temperature of 195° F

39. As part of the dishwashing inspection process, the dietary manager notices that many of the glasses have a film on them, which is most likely caused by:
    a. The hardness of the water
    b. The alkalinity of the water
    c. Inadequate use of detergent
    d. Improper glass placement within the dish machine

40. All of the following statements about the Safety Data Sheet (SDS) are true EXCEPT:
    a. The Occupation Safety and Health Administration requires that all employers must identify potential chemical hazards to its employees; in addition SDS must be kept on file relative to these chemicals
    b. The SDS should include physical and chemical properties of each chemical
    c. The SDS should include information about fire and explosive hazards
    d. Each employee must be given a copy of the SDS each year

41. A dietary manager is developing a standardized recipe at a nursing home based on a recipe from one of the residents. The recipe yield is for 4 servings, but 75 servings are needed to feed all of the residents. What factor is used to increase the recipe to provide the necessary number of servings?
    a. 0.053
    b. 300
    c. 18.75
    d. 20

42. A standard recipe calls for a basic veloute sauce, which is a:
    a. White sauce made by preparing a roux then adding hot milk to it
    b. White sauce made by preparing a roux then adding hot broth to it
    c. Sauce made by adding equal parts brown stock and brown sauce
    d. Brown sauce made by simmering beef bones, meat, and vegetables

43. What gauge stainless steel is appropriate for a 2½ quart sauce pan at a nursing home?
    a. 10
    b. 14
    c. 18
    d. 22

44. All of the following are acceptable ways to gather customer satisfaction information from nursing home residents EXCEPT for:
    a. Comment cards delivered on the food trays
    b. Plate waste studies
    c. Written surveys
    d. Secretly listening to conversations in the dining room

45. Colder than normal weather has affected certain crops in Florida, including tomatoes, strawberries, and citrus fruits. How might this knowledge affect the menu planning if a nursing home uses a 3-week menu cycle?
    a. Substitute other seasonal fruits for citrus or strawberries
    b. Omit salads from the menu because tomatoes may not be available
    c. Wait until prices start to increase to buy citrus fruits, strawberries, and tomatoes
    d. Change to a static menu

46. Which of the following statements best describes the inventory process?
    a. A perpetual inventory is the best way to keep track of what items are on hand
    b. A physical inventory is the best way to keep track of what items are on hand
    c. Tight inventory control is required to keep carrying costs down, thus saving money in the long term
    d. A tightly controlled inventory is not as important as keeping plenty of items on hand to prevent having to buy missing items at the last minute

47. A recipe for meatloaf calls for 80% lean ground beef. The portion size is 3 ounces, and 225 portions are needed. How much ground beef must be ordered?
    a. 37.5 pounds
    b. 42 pounds
    c. 84 pounds
    d. 57 pounds

48. To determine the price of beef stew being offered in the cafeteria, the dietary manager first determines what it costs to make the recipe then a markup is added. This is known as:
    a. Conventional pricing
    b. Demand-oriented pricing
    c. Prime-cost pricing
    d. Estimated pricing

49. If Mary works 20 hours a week, Stan works 16 hours a week on the weekends, Robert and Tim work 40 hours a week, and Stephanie works 32 hours a week, how many full-time equivalents (FTEs) are there?
    a. 148 FTEs
    b. 18.5 FTEs
    c. 3.7 FTEs
    d. 5 FTEs

50. A current steam table is old and breaks down often. A new table will typically be bought using money from which of the following accounts?
    a. Cash
    b. Capital
    c. Master
    d. Equipment

Answers and explanations

1. C: A medical record is a legal document. Any communication within this document must adhere to accepted standards and meet certain requirements. This includes month, day, year, and time of entry. Back dating and dating the entry ahead of time are illegal and unethical. If an error does occur, a single line is drawn in pen through the error accompanied by a note explaining the reason for the correction. The initials of the person making the correction and the date are also noted. The corrected information is then added to the record. The same procedure should be followed for electronic medical records except that all notations are done electronically. Care should be taken to make sure that hard copies of the record are also corrected. Correction fluid (White Out) and labels to cover the error are never used.

2. B: Generally accepted methods for obtaining a diet history include a 24-hour recall, a food frequency questionnaire, or a 3-day food record. Longer food records such as a 7-day food diary is helpful in certain situations but is not typically used with new nursing home residents. A food diary and food records record exactly what a person eats and drinks; however, the person must be capable of keeping this information, which is often a difficult task for a resident entering a nursing home. A food frequency questionnaire determines how often a person eats various types of foods, such as fruits, vegetables, dairy products, or protein sources, to look for potential nutrient deficiencies. A 24-hour recall determines what the person has consumed within the previous 24 hours. Often a family member is needed to obtain appropriate information.

3. A: The main purpose of nutrition screening is to identify individuals at risk for malnutrition. The screening tool used should be simple, fast, and effective in determining if risk factors are present. Parts of the screening process include obtaining anthropometric measurements, such as height, weight, and body mass index. Determining if any unintentional weight loss has occurred is also important. Other important information includes changes in the ability to chew, activity levels, appetite, and financial resources. Nutrition screening identifies individuals who require a nutritional assessment by a registered dietitian.

4. A: An elevated serum sodium level is the laboratory value that would most likely indicate dehydration. The normal range for serum sodium is 135–145 mEq/L. The serum potassium and albumin levels listed in the question are both within normal range and are unlikely to indicate dehydration. Other signs of dehydration include excessive thirst, a dry mouth, and decreased urine output. The appearance of urine would also be very concentrated, yellow, and malodorous. Other symptoms of dehydration include eyes that appear to be sunken, reduced tear output, decreased blood pressure, and increased heart rate. A rule of thumb for calculating fluid requirements for older adults is 30 mL/kg. This would mean the fluid requirements for a person weighing 50 kg (or 110 pounds) is 1500 mL/day or approximately 50 ounces.

5. D: When a person has diverticular disease, a high-fiber diet is recommended; however, if an inflammation occurs, such as diverticulitis, a low-fiber diet is indicated until the inflammation is resolved. A low-fiber diet removes foods that contain large amounts of fiber. Foods that should be avoided are whole-grain breads, cereals, pastas, and rice;

- 115 -

popcorn; raw vegetables; dried fruits; baked beans; dried beans; and nuts. Foods allowed on a low-fiber diet include white bread, pasta, and rice. Cereals should contain less than 1 gram of fiber for each serving. In this menu, the all-bran cereal would contain approximately 10 grams of fiber. Canned fruits and vegetables would be appropriate as well as fruits and vegetables without skins, seeds, or membranes. Dairy products are allowed as well as most protein sources.

6. C: The best lunch menu for the Muslin resident of the health care facility is meatloaf made from ground beef, mashed potatoes, steamed carrots, unsweetened canned pears, and low-fat milk. This would be soft enough to meet the requirements for mechanical soft, protein, and it eliminates concentrated sweets, such as tapioca pudding or ginger ale. Since the resident is Muslim, Islamic dietary restrictions must be taken into account, such as avoiding alcohol, pork, and pork products. All meat must be slaughtered in a way that removes all blood, and the meat must be well done. Hotdogs are usually a pork product, and meatballs are often a mix of beef, pork, and sometimes lamb. It is important to honor religious or ethnic food practices and to be culturally sensitive to all residents.

7. B: The Minimum Data Set (MDS) is the name of the form that is used for the assessment of nutrition. A care plan must be implemented within 7 days after the assessment of nutrition is completed. Usually the registered dietitian or the dietary manager completes the nutrition section of the MDS, which is section K. This section includes information about anthropometrics, nutrient intake, use of enteral or parenteral nutrition, and problems with nutrient intake, such as appetite changes or chewing issues. The care plans for all residents need to be updated quarterly. The resident described in the question is presently due for a follow-up. The care plan needs to include objectives that can be measured, such as weight maintained at the current level, and a time frame stating when interventions are needed and re-evaluation is necessary.

8. C: The guidelines state that the nutritional care plan should be updated quarterly or if a change in condition occurs. In this case, the fact that Mary is refusing meals and losing weight warrants immediate intervention. Objectives need to be written in such a way that outcomes can be measured and evaluated. A timetable must also be defined for determining if the intervention is effective. In Mary's case, an intervention may be to ask the physician to change her diet order to high calorie, high protein and initiate nutritional supplements, such as Ensure or Boost, twice a day between meals with weekly weight checks and follow-up. Mary's calorie intake can be recorded by the nursing staff. The measurable outcome would be that Mary meets at least 75% of her calorie requirements and that she regains her admission weight within 1 month.

9. C: A semiselective menu would be the best choice based on the size of the facility (75 beds) and the need to incorporate different dietary restrictions. A semiselective menu offers more than one choice in a few of the menu categories, such as entrees or desserts. This type of menu helps to control costs while allowing some options. A selective menu offers two or more choices for all categories listed on the menu. There are disadvantages to a full selective menu, such as production, inventory, and staffing requirements, but it does offer a full set of choices to the residents. A nonselective menu does not offer choice, but usually alternative selections are available so these ingredients must always be on hand. A static menu is a set menu that does not change from day to day. For longer lengths of stay, variety and choice become an issue.

10. D: Providing the wife with some simple information that covers the different types of fat in the diet from the American Heart Association could be the first step. Other sources for reputable nutrition education materials include the American Dietetic Association, MyPlate from the United States Department of Agriculture, the National Dairy Council, and the American Diabetes Association. Care must be taken when obtaining information randomly on the Internet as some web sites may not be accurate or appropriate. Providing information about reducing sodium in the diet is not really addressing the woman's request. Telling the woman that you are too busy does not send the best message about the quality of care her husband may be receiving, your commitment to nutrition, or your overall caring attitude.

11. B: A short-term hospital stay can be a good time to educate someone about dietary issues associated with chronic diseases, such as diabetes. An initial interview should elicit information regarding usual diet at home, previous diet education, and a history of the current disease, such as blood glucose records and medication use. After the initial education has occurred, using the menu as a teaching tool is very useful. Allowing the patient to select menu choices then reviewing them with him can be an effective way to teach the patient how to make good choices. Keeping a food record may also be helpful to assess snacking and food brought from home. The dietary manager can also ask open-ended questions that require an answer other than yes or no to assess comprehension. The patient should be involved in goal setting as it is more likely that compliance will occur. The involvement of the family is also helpful.

12. A: All residents need to be treated with respect and dignity regardless of the diet that has been ordered for them. Extra care must be taken for those who have difficulty chewing and swallowing and require a texture-modified diet, such as puree or minced food. These texture modifications can be quite unappealing, and steps must be taken to ensure variety in color, food choices, and flavor. The USDA's MyPlate should be used if possible in planning meals to ensure all nutrient requirements are met. Pureeing the menu items is possible but should only be done if the results are acceptable. Certain foods are not appropriate for pureeing, such as celery, which is too stringy. Foods should also be precooked in a way to maximize nutrition and ease of altering the texture. Acceptable seasonings should be used. The use of plates with dividers is also a good way to help with presentation and keep the various foods separate.

13. B: Enteral products are generally commercially prepared products that are provided either orally or through a tube. Sometimes facilities prepare their own enteral products. These are typically used for patients who are not able to meet nutritional requirements on their own. Oral nutritional supplements are often used for patients who are experiencing weight loss, and a key marker is 5% weight loss in a 1-month period. As a result of cost constraints, a patient who is requesting milkshakes can often be offered a less expensive alternative. A person on a "no concentrated sweets" diet may receive supplements if indicated but may require a low-carbohydrate option. A patient who is having difficulty swallowing may need intervention by a speech pathologist before supplements are implemented to assess swallowing function.

14. D: Continuous Quality Improvement is a management practice that looks at the organization and its systems as a way to improve quality. Plate waste studies measure the amount of food left on the plate after the meal is completed. This type of study can help to determine if food is acceptable, if certain recipes are acceptable, or the overall waste of a

certain meal. Patient surveys are a way to get the opinions of patients. The survey can be designed in a way that asks questions about specific food items with a scale to rate them or the food service/food quality as a whole. A test tray is a sample tray sent to the patient area that is then tested for temperature, quality, and taste, by a manager or supervisor. Employee surveys can be useful in some situations but not when patient input is needed.

15. C: A patient satisfaction survey is a way to obtain the opinion of the patient on various aspects of the food service operation. It can also be used for benchmarking purposes where the information obtained can be compared to information obtained by other facilities of similar size and scope. Information is obtained with questions pertaining to variety, portion size, temperature, timing of meals, quality of service provided by the food service employees, and tray or menu accuracy. The questions are often tied to a scale where patients indicate their selection with a range of very poor or extremely dissatisfied to excellent or extremely satisfied. Information on the opinion of cost is not usually obtained because this information is not widely available to patients. Many times, an open-ended question or statement is included where any information that has not already been provided can be written.

16. B: Portion control is a very important function in food service. It helps with cost control, patient or customer satisfaction, and quality control. Food is portioned in many different ways: by weight, such as ounces for protein; by count, such as fresh fruit or individual rolls; or standard serving sizes, such as by scoop, dipper, or ladle. Scoops or dippers are available in sizes of 6 to 100. A rule of thumb is the larger the number of the scoop size, the smaller the portion. For example, a #100 scoop is equal to 2 teaspoons. A #6 scoop is equal to two-thirds cup. A #8 scoop is equal to one-half cup and would be the appropriate selection to serve one-half cup of mashed potatoes. Ladles are used for liquid foods and range from 1 to 12 ounces.

17. B: One full-time equivalent (FTE) is equal to a 40-hour work week. Based on the above scenario, three people are full-time employees who work 40 hours each (3 FTEs), and 10 employees work 20 hours a week, which is 5 FTEs (0.5 FTEs each). Six employees work 24 hours a week at 0.6 FTEs each or 3.6 FTEs total, and one person works on weekends only for 16 hours or 0.4 FTE. The total number of FTEs is 12. Many schedules involve a varying number of full- and part-time employees, and FTEs help to control labor costs and to develop a more efficient schedule. It enables food service and other businesses to adopt a schedule that best fits their needs and maximizes productive time. It is not good business practice to have all employees scheduled during times where there is not much to be done.

18. C: A job description is a document that should be written and available for all positions within an organization. This typically lists the job title, job code, and the location of the position. It also lists a summary of the duties and responsibilities of the specific position as well as any special skills and qualifications needed. The job description should also specify to whom the employee reports and if other employees must be supervised. A job specification is similar but is geared more toward outlining the minimum standards or requirements that must be met to qualify for a certain position. For example, it may list a physical requirement of the ability to lift 40 pounds. It may specify educational requirements, such as the ability to read, write, and converse in English. A job analysis breaks the job down into individual tasks and assigns a timeline for each.

19. D: There are federal and state laws in place that protect against discrimination on the basis of race, skin color, ethnicity, religion, gender, age, marital status, pregnancy, or having a family. Employers should also not ask about sexual preference, disabilities, or status as a U.S. citizen. Employers may ask if the person being interviewed is authorized to work in the country. Of all the questions listed in the question, the one commenting on the engagement ring is unacceptable because it is an indirect way of finding out about wedding plans. It could also be an indirect way of inferring that one may be starting a family soon, which may influence hiring decisions.

20. C: Termination is not generally an initial response to poor employee performance unless there is a safety or other serious issue, such as illegal drug use. If the employee is new or if the issue has just developed, it is reasonable to sit down with the employee and review the overall job description. A discussion involving the employee's role in making sure mistakes are not present on each tray sets the minimum performance standard. A performance improvement plan is a formal way to address areas that need improvement by an employee. It helps to delineate expectations and to assist with change so as to achieve the expectations set. Corrective action is a process that addresses, documents, and corrects issues with an employee. It normally involves a verbal warning followed by a written warning then suspension and finally termination if the issue is not corrected.

21. A: The Age Discrimination in Employment Act of 1967 was the original law that protected workers and job applicants age 40 and older from discrimination based on age. This law was amended in 1990 to stop employers from denying or cancelling benefits to older workers. The amendment is called the Older Workers Benefit Protection Act of 1990. The law includes protection to those who are seeking to enter an apprenticeship program. It protects workers against harassment based on age. This law is administered by the United States Equal Employment Opportunity Commission.

22. B: The Food and Drug Administration (FDA) has written and published the Food Code that helps keep the food supply safe, especially food served at food service establishments. It is a set of rules and regulations to guide those responsible for food production. In the four scenarios listed in the question, the one involving home-baked zucchini bread would be in direct violation of the FDA Food Code mainly because it was produced in a private home. Only food produced in a facility that complies with the law may be sold or served. The FDA Food Code deals with other areas, such as equipment, utensils, linens, toxic materials, and waste processing. It also deals with physical facilities, such as the material used for floors or the use of light bulbs. The FDA Food Code deals with the health of employees, personal hygiene, and behavior in the work area, such as eating or drinking. It is a comprehensive document that is updated every few years.

23. C: A participative management style is one where management seeks input from the employees and allows employees to participate in the decision-making process. The idea is that if employees take ownership of issues, outcomes may improve. An authoritative style is based on following rules and does not welcome input from employees. A proactive management style is one where the manager acts on issues before they blow up and become major problems. An autocratic style is one where employees do exactly what they are told to do when they are told to do it. The manager likes to be in complete control. Autocratic style does not motivate employees as well as a participative or proactive style may.

24. D: The Health Insurance Portability and Accountability Act of 1996 was written to provide protection and privacy to all personal health information. This includes how health information is discussed by others, transmitted, and processed. It applies to all health insurance companies and to facilities and personnel who provide health care, such as hospitals, clinics, doctors, and nurses. All information that is entered into a medical record is protected as well as any discussions with a health care provider or information that can be obtained in the computer. There are procedures in place to make everyone aware of this law and to disclose how this is accomplished. It also governs who can access health information. Employees are required to attend periodic retraining on the law.

25. C: The actual codes for local and state health departments vary from state to state, but following standard food safety practices as a department goal should yield acceptable results. The danger zone for food is considered to be between 40°F and 140°F. Any temperature within this range raises the risk of bacterial contamination. Thawing foods is one way that temperatures can enter this zone; however, thawing food in the refrigerator lessens this risk if it is at the proper temperature of 40°F. Raw meat is always a potential source of contamination and storing it above fresh produce is not practicing proper food safety and may result in a potential citation. Hazard Analysis and Critical Control Points is a system where a plan is put in place for making sure all aspects of food service are safe at all points in the spectrum. This includes shipping, receiving, storage, production, and service.

26. D: A dietary manager interacts with many professionals, including physicians, nurses, dietitians, and therapists, in most jobs. They are considered part of the health care team and may often notice issues that may not have been addressed. Referrals can be made through the nurse or physician on the suggestion of a dietary manager. One example may be a change in the ability of a patient or resident to eat. Aspiration is a serious issue and may present as drooling, pocketing food, coughing or gagging when trying to swallow, vomiting after meals, or being afraid to eat. If any of these signs are noticed in a long-term care facility, a referral to a speech therapist is warranted to check for possible aspiration and to put a plan in place to address the problem if it is present. Other types of referral may be to congregate meals, elder services, or support groups.

27. A: Federal requirements for nursing homes address many different issues. One of the issues addressed is the timing of meals. Residents must be provided with three meals a day of attractive and nutritious food. No more than 14 hours can pass from the last large meal of the evening until breakfast the next morning. If a nourishing snack is provided, such as cheese and crackers or a sandwich, the time between meals can stretch to 16 hours. In the scenarios listed in the question, if dinner is served at 5 p.m. and breakfast is served at 9 a.m., 16 hours have passed, and an evening snack has not been provided. The easiest solution is to provide a nourishing evening snack around 8 p.m. This shortens the time between nourishing meals to 13 hours, which is well within federal guidelines. It is also the least disruptive to overall food service scheduling.

28. B: Federal regulations require that all nursing homes regardless of the state in which they are located must employ the services of a registered dietitian (RD). A RD has successfully completed requirements of the Commission on Dietetic Registration. Many states also require RDs to be licensed. The nursing home must be sure they are indeed hiring a person with the correct qualification who can be hired as a full-time, part-time, or consulting dietitian. In all of these cases, the dietitian must have frequent contact with the

director of food services. A food service director cannot function as a dietitian without the proper qualifications.

29. B: The United States Department of Agriculture inspects and grades meat, poultry, eggs, fruits, vegetables, and dairy products. The grades available for poultry are US Grades A, B, and C. The grades are based on the amount of fat and skin and the presence of defects. Meats are graded based on US Prime, Choice, Select, or Standard. Eggs are graded using US Grades AA, A, and B. Fresh fruits and vegetables are graded using US Fancy, Extra No. 1, No. 1, and No. 2, or Combination. Canned fruits and vegetables are graded using US Grade A, B, C, or D.

30. D: A Select cut of meat indicates it has less marbling than Choice and Prime cuts and may, therefore, be less tender and less flavorful. Pan frying, grilling, and oven roasting may produce a less tender product unless the cut is from the loin or rib. Other Select cuts may need to be marinated first to obtain a tender product. Braising would be the preferable method of cooking a Select cut. Prime grade is the most flavorful, contains the most marbling, and can be cooked using dry methods, such as roasting, grilling, or broiling. The choice grade is just below Prime and contains less marbling and is not as tender as the Prime grade. Dry cooking methods can be used as long as the meat is not overcooked. Braising methods can also be used. Less preferred grades include Standard or Commercial, and Utility, Cutter, and Canner.

31. B: Food should never be stored on the floor. Instead, shelves, pallets, or some other type of platform should be used so the food is stored above the floor. Metal shelves are the type typically used for storing food. Air should be able to flow freely around the shelves for circulation. Any type of dry food that has been opened, such as rice, pasta, flour, or sugar, should be stored in a container with a tight-fitting lid to preserve freshness. It is appropriate that the food just delivered is being placed at the back of the shelf. This is done so the product that has been there the longest is used first. This is called the first in, first out.

32. C: There are guidelines available for the maximum length of time various foods can be stored. Fresh meat, poultry, milk, dairy products, and eggs must be kept at a temperature between 32°F and 40°F. Fresh poultry stored longer than 2 days must be discarded. Ground beef can be kept at the appropriate temperature for up to 2 days. Storage times for dairy products vary, depending on the product. Milk can be stored for 3 days, butter for 2 weeks, and eggs in the shell for 3 weeks. Fresh fish should typically be used within 2 days, and shellfish, within 5 days. These are just guidelines, and the actual time for storage depends on conditions, temperature, and the product itself.

33. C: *Escherichia coli* (commonly known as *E. coli*) infection can be spread through water contaminated with cow feces or through contaminated food, such as undercooked ground beef. It can also be contracted through contaminated swimming pools. Day care centers can also be a source as a result of the large number of dirty diapers and the need for frequent hand washing. Symptoms can present around 7 days after consuming the bacteria. The most common symptoms of *E. coli* infection are bloody diarrhea and abdominal cramping. Fever is not always present. In some cases, this illness can lead to complications, such as hemolytic uremic syndrome, which can cause kidney failure. Diagnosis is through a stool culture taken within 48 hours after symptoms present.

34. A: Any time a certain disease is discovered, the local health department should be notified either by the physician who has diagnosed it or the laboratory where the test was conducted. This would include reporting food-borne illness caused by *Escherichia coli*, *Salmonella*, or *Campylobacter*. Other diseases that need to be reported include tuberculosis and hepatitis. The local health department will report to the state health department and, eventually, to the Centers for Disease Control. The state health department tracks the diseases that are reported. Any time multiple reports are received, an investigation occurs to identify the cause of the outbreak.

35. B: Roast beef evenly cooked to a medium rare temperature of 145°F is least likely to cause a food-borne illness when compared to the other choices listed in the question. A roast comes from one animal and is not processed like ground beef, which is more likely to cause illness if eaten rare (or even medium rare). Raw eggs and raw shellfish are likely to cause food-borne illness. Fresh fruits and vegetables can also cause food-borne illness as a result of inadequate washing, using impure water to rinse, or the use of cow manure for fertilizer. If eaten fresh, the item does not undergo cooking, this effectively kills any bacteria present. Alfalfa sprouts pose a significant high risk and are not allowed under the Food and Drug Administration Food Code. Unpasteurized juices and milk are also a risk and should be avoided.

36. D: There are four main points that will help employees remember steps to prevent food-borne illness. The first is cleaning; frequent hand washing, using warm water and soap for at least 20 seconds, is a necessity. This must be done before any food is handled as well as after. Surfaces, such as cutting boards and counters, should always be scrubbed with hot soapy water before food is prepared as well as after. All fresh produce should be rinsed well under clean running water. The second point is to separate surfaces. Raw meat and produce must be prepared separately, using separate cutting boards and knives. The third point is cooking food thoroughly. A food thermometer must be used to ensure cooked food reaches the appropriate internal temperature. The fourth point is proper chilling. Foods must be refrigerated within 4 hours if not eaten right away. Large quantities of food need to be placed in shallow containers so the food cools quickly.

37. B: OSHA stands for Occupational Safety and Health Administration. It is part of the United States Department of Labor. The main function of OSHA is maintaining a safe work environment for all. OSHA requires the use of safety or personal protective equipment for certain employees who are doing specific types of jobs. It also requires careful record-keeping of any accident or incident for the purpose of investigating and implementing the appropriate action. It keeps statistics on the rate of injury and different types of inspection results. OSHA has many safety guidelines dealing with a wide range of topics from alcohol in the workplace to hazardous waste removal to pyrotechnics to welding safety. OSHA does a lot of different types of training and publishes a wide range of publications for employers, employees, and the general public. The function of OSHA is wide ranging but deals mainly with keeping employees safe in the workplace.

38. C: There are two types of dish washing machines for commercial use. These are hot water sanitizing or chemical sanitizing, using either a solution of chlorine, iodine, or quaternary ammonium solution. The minimum water temperature during the wash cycle for a conveyor, dual temperature machine is 160°F. The maximum temperature for a hot water sanitizing rinse is 195°F. Any temperature hotter than this will cause the water to evaporate quickly and will not provide sufficient sanitizing. For chemical sanitizing

machines using a chlorine solution, the final rinse temperature should be 120°F. When inspecting a dish machine, at least two complete wash and rinse cycles must be done before an accurate temperature reading can be taken. The temperatures should be measured directly from the tanks.

39. A: There are many issues that can arise in the dishwashing process. If a film or spotting is seen on glasses or plates, the hardness of the water may be the cause. Installing a water softener or the use of a chlorinated detergent may help with this issue. Also, the temperature of both the wash and rinse cycles should be checked. Film can also be due to water temperatures being too high. Other potential issues with dishwashing could be streaking, which may be caused by the alkaline level of the water being too high. If dishes are coming out dirty, the detergent should be checked as well as the water temperatures for the wash and rinse cycles. Dirty dishes may also be result from the incorrect placement of the dishes in the machine.

40. D: SDS stands for Safety Data Sheet. It is an OSHA regulation that all workplaces must have on file a SDS for each potentially hazardous chemical located on site. The SDS should contain information about each chemical, including physical and chemical properties, potential health hazards, information on reactivity, and potential fire and explosive hazards. The SDS also includes information of the safe use of the product and how the product is handled and stored. Other information includes necessary protective equipment, limits on exposure to the chemical, and information regarding emergency care or first-aid treatment. The standard format for the SDS has sixteen sections; all relevant information should be included within.

41. C: The factor that would be used to increase the number of servings from 4 to 75 would be 18.75. Standardized recipes are used in food service establishments to help control quality, and a computerized program can easily help to accomplish this. Other benefits to standardized recipes are that a recipe can be specifically adapted for the effective use of the facility's equipment and personnel as well as to provide a consistent product to customers. The consistency aspect would involve standard ingredients, portion size, and outcome. The product should turn out the same way each time it is prepared. Standardized recipes include a title, recipe yield, portion size, temperature, length of time needed to cook, the ingredients, and amounts. It also includes the procedure for preparing the recipe.

42. B: In food production, recipe terms have standard definitions that are generally accepted by all who prepare food. When a cook reads or prepares a recipe, he or she should instinctively know to what the term is referring. A veloute sauce is a type of white sauce that is made by preparing a roux then adding hot broth. A béchamel sauce is similar except it uses hot milk as the liquid. A roux is equal parts of flour and butter cooked together for a certain length of time, depending on whether it is for a white or brown sauce. Roux is used for thickening. A basic white sauce is the basis for many sauces and gravies and can be modified as needed by adding various ingredients, such as cheeses or spices.

43. C: The gauge of metal specifies the weight of the metal but not thickness. In general, if the gauge is a low number, it is a heavier metal. Saucepans are usually made from 18–20 gauge metal. Heavier gauges are not as conducive to cooking as they do not conduct heat as well. A specification also includes the name of the product to be purchased, specific size or dimensions of the product, materials, and how it is constructed. The specification may also

include price and delivery data. Other items may have safety requirements specified by certain groups, such as Underwriters Laboratories or American Standards Association.

44. D: Addressing customer or patient satisfaction is an important management function. There are many ways to obtain the necessary information, much of which is subjective. Customer comment cards can be delivered to the patient or made available at various locations. Written or oral surveys can be conducted. Sales data can be used to evaluate data over time, looking for trends, such as a decrease in ordering of macaroni and cheese after the recipe changed. Frequency ratings are another way to assess satisfaction where customers can assign rankings to certain menu items when asked. Plate waste studies are another technique to observe what is being consumed and what is being thrown out. Informal discussions with customers are another way to assess satisfaction; however, it should not be done secretly. If a conversation happens to be overheard, one could step in and ask for clarification and try to address concerns on the spot.

45. A: Forecasting is predicting how much food you need for a day or a certain amount of time. Many factors affect forecasting and menu planning. Certainly the weather is a big factor. If the cold weather has affected certain crops in Florida, such as citrus fruits, strawberries, and tomatoes, dietary managers will likely run into trouble with availability or prohibitive costs. It would be a wise decision to address the issue before it becomes a problem. Substitutions would be an appropriate step to take. Omitting salads may not be a reasonable option as many people enjoy salads. Perhaps altering the salad composition is an option by reducing the number of tomatoes or by finding an alternative source. Waiting for prices to increase would certainly affect the budget and would not be a wise decision, given that the knowledge was available beforehand.

46. C: Inventory is a very important part of the functioning of a food service operation. Keeping a tightly controlled inventory helps to keep carrying costs down as these costs can run as high as 40% or 50% of the value of the inventory. Fast food restaurants have lower carrying costs because the inventory turns over rapidly. A physical inventory is a manual count of all items on hand, and a perpetual inventory is a master inventory level that is adjusted on paper each time items are used. Often times, perpetual inventories are computerized. Typically, a combination of both methods is used to keep inventories accurate and controlled. It is important to try to keep items on hand for when they are needed but at levels that ensure the items are used before they expire.

47. D: Determining how much product to buy for a recipe is dependent on a number of factors, including edible portion, portion size, number of servings required, and as purchased product. In the example above, 1 pound of 80% lean ground beef has an approximate yield of 0.74 pounds. Because it contains fat and shrinks during cooking, only a portion of the ground beef is considered edible. For 225 3-ounce portions, 675 ounces of ground beef are needed, or 42.2 pounds. This number is divided by the yield of 0.74; thus, approximately 57 pounds of 80% lean ground beef is needed to make the meatloaf recipe.

48. A: There are many ways to determine the cost of a menu item. Conventional pricing determines what it costs to make the recipe (called raw food cost), and then a markup is added to cover incidentals, such as salt, pepper, and napkins, after which an additional profit markup is added. Demand-oriented pricing uses a model that estimates what customers are willing to pay for an item, and the price is set according to this. For example, it may cost only $1 a portion to make macaroni and cheese; however, customers are willing

to pay $4 for a serving because it is a quality product. Prime-cost pricing takes into account both labor and raw food cost. Items are priced differently based on the degree of difficulty of the preparation.

49. C: A full-time equivalent is equal to 40 hours. One person working 40 hours a week will equal 1 FTE as will two employees each working 20 hours a week. The above example has five employees working a total of 148 hours a week. To determine the number of FTEs, 148 hours is divided by 40 hours to get 3.7 FTEs. It does not technically matter how many employees there are, but rather, the number of hours that need to be covered. Many places of employment offer part-time work to employees and, thus, do not have to offer certain benefits, such as retirement benefits, which saves the company money. Other companies only hire full-time employees.

50. B: The capital account is the account from which money for expensive items is taken. This type of account covers long-term needs, such as replacement of worn out equipment and remodeling projects. The cash account contains cash on hand to cover expenditures. The operating account incorporates money for running an establishment, such as labor, food costs, supplies, electricity, heat, and any other overhead items, such as building costs. The master account incorporates all aspects of spending, including cash, capital, and operating expenses.

Secret Key #1 - Time is Your Greatest Enemy

Pace Yourself

Wear a watch. At the beginning of the test, check the time (or start a chronometer on your watch to count the minutes), and check the time after every few questions to make sure you are "on schedule."

If you are forced to speed up, do it efficiently. Usually one or more answer choices can be eliminated without too much difficulty. Above all, don't panic. Don't speed up and just begin guessing at random choices. By pacing yourself, and continually monitoring your progress against your watch, you will always know exactly how far ahead or behind you are with your available time. If you find that you are one minute behind on the test, don't skip one question without spending any time on it, just to catch back up. Take 15 fewer seconds on the next four questions, and after four questions you'll have caught back up. Once you catch back up, you can continue working each problem at your normal pace.

Furthermore, don't dwell on the problems that you were rushed on. If a problem was taking up too much time and you made a hurried guess, it must be difficult. The difficult questions are the ones you are most likely to miss anyway, so it isn't a big loss. It is better to end with more time than you need than to run out of time.

Lastly, sometimes it is beneficial to slow down if you are constantly getting ahead of time. You are always more likely to catch a careless mistake by working more slowly than quickly, and among very high-scoring test takers (those who are likely to have lots of time left over), careless errors affect the score more than mastery of material.

Secret Key #2 - Guessing is not Guesswork

You probably know that guessing is a good idea. Unlike other standardized tests, there is no penalty for getting a wrong answer. Even if you have no idea about a question, you still have a 20-25% chance of getting it right.

Most test takers do not understand the impact that proper guessing can have on their score. Unless you score extremely high, guessing will significantly contribute to your final score.

Monkeys Take the Test

What most test takers don't realize is that to insure that 20-25% chance, you have to guess randomly. If you put 20 monkeys in a room to take this test, assuming they answered once per question and behaved themselves, on average they would get 20-25% of the questions correct. Put 20 test takers in the room, and the average will be much lower among guessed questions. Why?

1. The test writers intentionally write deceptive answer choices that "look" right. A test taker has no idea about a question, so he picks the "best looking" answer, which is often wrong. The monkey has no idea what looks good and what doesn't, so it will consistently be right about 20-25% of the time.

2. Test takers will eliminate answer choices from the guessing pool based on a hunch or intuition. Simple but correct answers often get excluded, leaving a 0% chance of being correct. The monkey has no clue, and often gets lucky with the best choice.

This is why the process of elimination endorsed by most test courses is flawed and detrimental to your performance. Test takers don't guess; they make an ignorant stab in the dark that is usually worse than random.

$5 Challenge

Let me introduce one of the most valuable ideas of this course—the $5 challenge:

You only mark your "best guess" if you are willing to bet $5 on it.
You only eliminate choices from guessing if you are willing to bet $5 on it.

Why $5? Five dollars is an amount of money that is small yet not insignificant, and can really add up fast (20 questions could cost you $100). Likewise, each answer choice on one question of the test will have a small impact on your overall score, but it can really add up to a lot of points in the end.

The process of elimination IS valuable. The following shows your chance of guessing it right:

If you eliminate wrong answer choices until only this many remain:	Chance of getting it correct:
1	100%
2	50%
3	33%

However, if you accidentally eliminate the right answer or go on a hunch for an incorrect answer, your chances drop dramatically—to 0%. By guessing among all the answer choices, you are GUARANTEED to have a shot at the right answer.

That's why the $5 test is so valuable. If you give up the advantage and safety of a pure guess, it had better be worth the risk.

What we still haven't covered is how to be sure that whatever guess you make is truly random. Here's the easiest way:

Always pick the first answer choice among those remaining.

Such a technique means that you have decided, **before you see a single test question**, exactly how you are going to guess, and since the order of choices tells you nothing about which one is correct, this guessing technique is perfectly random.

This section is not meant to scare you away from making educated guesses or eliminating choices; you just need to define when a choice is worth eliminating. The $5 test, along with a pre-defined random guessing strategy, is the best way to make sure you reap all of the benefits of guessing.

Secret Key #3 - Practice Smarter, Not Harder

Many test takers delay the test preparation process because they dread the awful amounts of practice time they think necessary to succeed on the test. We have refined an effective method that will take you only a fraction of the time.

There are a number of "obstacles" in the path to success. Among these are answering questions, finishing in time, and mastering test-taking strategies. All must be executed on the day of the test at peak performance, or your score will suffer. The test is a mental marathon that has a large impact on your future.

Just like a marathon runner, it is important to work your way up to the full challenge. So first you just worry about questions, and then time, and finally strategy:

Success Strategy

1. Find a good source for practice tests.
2. If you are willing to make a larger time investment, consider using more than one study guide. Often the different approaches of multiple authors will help you "get" difficult concepts.
3. Take a practice test with no time constraints, with all study helps, "open book." Take your time with questions and focus on applying strategies.
4. Take a practice test with time constraints, with all guides, "open book."
5. Take a final practice test without open material and with time limits.

If you have time to take more practice tests, just repeat step 5. By gradually exposing yourself to the full rigors of the test environment, you will condition your mind to the stress of test day and maximize your success.

Secret Key #4 - Prepare, Don't Procrastinate

Let me state an obvious fact: if you take the test three times, you will probably get three different scores. This is due to the way you feel on test day, the level of preparedness you have, and the version of the test you see. Despite the test writers' claims to the contrary, some versions of the test WILL be easier for you than others.

Since your future depends so much on your score, you should maximize your chances of success. In order to maximize the likelihood of success, you've got to prepare in advance. This means taking practice tests and spending time learning the information and test taking strategies you will need to succeed.

Never go take the actual test as a "practice" test, expecting that you can just take it again if you need to. Take all the practice tests you can on your own, but when you go to take the official test, be prepared, be focused, and do your best the first time!

Secret Key #5 - Test Yourself

Everyone knows that time is money. There is no need to spend too much of your time or too little of your time preparing for the test. You should only spend as much of your precious time preparing as is necessary for you to get the score you need.

Once you have taken a practice test under real conditions of time constraints, then you will know if you are ready for the test or not.

If you have scored extremely high the first time that you take the practice test, then there is not much point in spending countless hours studying. You are already there.

Benchmark your abilities by retaking practice tests and seeing how much you have improved. Once you consistently score high enough to guarantee success, then you are ready.

If you have scored well below where you need, then knuckle down and begin studying in earnest. Check your improvement regularly through the use of practice tests under real conditions. Above all, don't worry, panic, or give up. The key is perseverance!

Then, when you go to take the test, remain confident and remember how well you did on the practice tests. If you can score high enough on a practice test, then you can do the same on the real thing.

General Strategies

The most important thing you can do is to ignore your fears and jump into the test immediately. Do not be overwhelmed by any strange-sounding terms. You have to jump into the test like jumping into a pool—all at once is the easiest way.

Make Predictions

As you read and understand the question, try to guess what the answer will be. Remember that several of the answer choices are wrong, and once you begin reading them, your mind will immediately become cluttered with answer choices designed to throw you off. Your mind is typically the most focused immediately after you have read the question and digested its contents. If you can, try to predict what the correct answer will be. You may be surprised at what you can predict.

Quickly scan the choices and see if your prediction is in the listed answer choices. If it is, then you can be quite confident that you have the right answer. It still won't hurt to check the other answer choices, but most of the time, you've got it!

Answer the Question

It may seem obvious to only pick answer choices that answer the question, but the test writers can create some excellent answer choices that are wrong. Don't pick an answer just because it sounds right, or you believe it to be true. It MUST answer the question. Once you've made your selection, always go back and check it against the question and make sure that you didn't misread the question and that the answer choice does answer the question posed.

Benchmark

After you read the first answer choice, decide if you think it sounds correct or not. If it doesn't, move on to the next answer choice. If it does, mentally mark that answer choice. This doesn't mean that you've definitely selected it as your answer choice, it just means that it's the best you've seen thus far. Go ahead and read the next choice. If the next choice is worse than the one you've already selected, keep going to the next answer choice. If the next choice is better than the choice you've already selected, mentally mark the new answer choice as your best guess.

The first answer choice that you select becomes your standard. Every other answer choice must be benchmarked against that standard. That choice is correct until proven otherwise by another answer choice beating it out. Once you've decided that no other answer choice seems as good, do one final check to ensure that your answer choice answers the question posed.

Valid Information

Don't discount any of the information provided in the question. Every piece of information may be necessary to determine the correct answer. None of the information in the question is there to throw you off (while the answer choices will certainly have information to throw you off). If two seemingly unrelated topics are discussed, don't ignore either. You can be confident there is a relationship, or it wouldn't be included in the question, and you are probably going to have to determine what is that relationship to find the answer.

Avoid "Fact Traps"

Don't get distracted by a choice that is factually true. Your search is for the answer that answers the question. Stay focused and don't fall for an answer that is true but irrelevant. Always go back to the question and make sure you're choosing an answer that actually answers the question and is not just a true statement. An answer can be factually correct, but it MUST answer the question asked. Additionally, two answers can both be seemingly correct, so be sure to read all of the answer choices, and make sure that you get the one that BEST answers the question.

Milk the Question

Some of the questions may throw you completely off. They might deal with a subject you have not been exposed to, or one that you haven't reviewed in years. While your lack of knowledge about the subject will be a hindrance, the question itself can give you many clues that will help you find the correct answer. Read the question carefully and look for clues. Watch particularly for adjectives and nouns describing difficult terms or words that you don't recognize. Regardless of whether you completely understand a word or not, replacing it with a synonym, either provided or one you more familiar with, may help you to understand what the questions are asking. Rather than wracking your mind about specific detailed information concerning a difficult term or word, try to use mental substitutes that are easier to understand.

The Trap of Familiarity

Don't just choose a word because you recognize it. On difficult questions, you may not recognize a number of words in the answer choices. The test writers don't put "make-believe" words on the test, so don't think that just because you only recognize all the words in one answer choice that that answer choice must be correct. If you only recognize words in one answer choice, then focus on that one. Is it correct? Try your best to determine if it is correct. If it is, that's great. If not, eliminate it. Each word and answer choice you eliminate increases your chances of getting the question correct, even if you then have to guess among the unfamiliar choices.

Eliminate Answers

Eliminate choices as soon as you realize they are wrong. But be careful! Make sure you consider all of the possible answer choices. Just because one appears right, doesn't mean that the next one won't be even better! The test writers will usually put more than one good answer choice for every question, so read all of them. Don't worry if you are stuck between two that seem right. By getting down to just two remaining possible choices, your odds are now 50/50. Rather than wasting too much time, play the odds. You are guessing, but guessing wisely because you've been able to knock out some of the answer choices that you know are wrong. If you are eliminating choices and realize that the last answer choice you are left with is also obviously wrong, don't panic. Start over and consider each choice again. There may easily be something that you missed the first time and will realize on the second pass.

Tough Questions

If you are stumped on a problem or it appears too hard or too difficult, don't waste time. Move on! Remember though, if you can quickly check for obviously incorrect answer choices, your chances of guessing correctly are greatly improved. Before you completely give up, at least try to knock out a couple of possible answers. Eliminate what you can and then guess at the remaining answer choices before moving on.

Brainstorm

If you get stuck on a difficult question, spend a few seconds quickly brainstorming. Run through the complete list of possible answer choices. Look at each choice and ask yourself, "Could this answer the question satisfactorily?" Go through each answer choice and consider it independently of the others. By systematically going through all possibilities, you may find something that you would otherwise overlook. Remember though that when you get stuck, it's important to try to keep moving.

Read Carefully

Understand the problem. Read the question and answer choices carefully. Don't miss the question because you misread the terms. You have plenty of time to read each question thoroughly and make sure you understand what is being asked. Yet a happy medium must be attained, so don't waste too much time. You must read carefully, but efficiently.

Face Value

When in doubt, use common sense. Always accept the situation in the problem at face value. Don't read too much into it. These problems will not require you to make huge leaps of logic. The test writers aren't trying to throw you off with a cheap trick. If you have to go beyond creativity and make a leap of logic in order to have an answer choice answer the question, then you should look at the other answer choices. Don't overcomplicate the problem by creating theoretical relationships or explanations that will warp time or space. These are normal problems rooted in reality. It's just that the applicable relationship or explanation may not be readily apparent and you have to figure things out. Use your common sense to interpret anything that isn't clear.

Prefixes

If you're having trouble with a word in the question or answer choices, try dissecting it. Take advantage of every clue that the word might include. Prefixes and suffixes can be a huge help. Usually they allow you to determine a basic meaning. Pre- means before, post- means after, pro - is positive, de- is negative. From these prefixes and suffixes, you can get an idea of the general meaning of the word and try to put it into context. Beware though of any traps. Just because con- is the opposite of pro-, doesn't necessarily mean congress is the opposite of progress!

Hedge Phrases

Watch out for critical hedge phrases, led off with words such as "likely," "may," "can," "sometimes," "often," "almost," "mostly," "usually," "generally," "rarely," and "sometimes." Question writers insert these hedge phrases to cover every possibility. Often an answer choice will be wrong simply because it leaves no room for exception. Unless the situation calls for them, avoid answer choices that have definitive words like "exactly," and "always."

Switchback Words

Stay alert for "switchbacks." These are the words and phrases frequently used to alert you to shifts in thought. The most common switchback word is "but." Others include "although," "however," "nevertheless," "on the other hand," "even though," "while," "in spite of," "despite," and "regardless of."

New Information

Correct answer choices will rarely have completely new information included. Answer choices typically are straightforward reflections of the material asked about and will directly relate to the question. If a new piece of information is included in an answer choice that doesn't even seem to relate to the topic being asked about, then that answer choice is likely incorrect. All of the information needed to answer the question is usually provided for you in the question. You should not have to make guesses that are unsupported or choose answer choices that require unknown information that cannot be reasoned from what is given.

Time Management

On technical questions, don't get lost on the technical terms. Don't spend too much time on any one question. If you don't know what a term means, then odds are you aren't going to get much further since you don't have a dictionary. You should be able to immediately recognize whether or not you know a term. If you don't, work with the other clues that you have—the other answer choices and terms provided—but don't waste too much time trying to figure out a difficult term that you don't know.

Contextual Clues

Look for contextual clues. An answer can be right but not the correct answer. The contextual clues will help you find the answer that is most right and is correct. Understand the context in which a phrase or statement is made. This will help you make important distinctions.

Don't Panic

Panicking will not answer any questions for you; therefore, it isn't helpful. When you first see the question, if your mind goes blank, take a deep breath. Force yourself to mechanically go through the steps of solving the problem using the strategies you've learned.

Pace Yourself

Don't get clock fever. It's easy to be overwhelmed when you're looking at a page full of questions, your mind is full of random thoughts and feeling confused, and the clock is ticking down faster than you would like. Calm down and maintain the pace that you have set for yourself. As long as you are on track by monitoring your pace, you are guaranteed to have enough time for yourself. When you get to the last few minutes of the test, it may seem like you won't have enough time left, but if you only have as many questions as you should have left at that point, then you're right on track!

Answer Selection

The best way to pick an answer choice is to eliminate all of those that are wrong, until only one is left and confirm that is the correct answer. Sometimes though, an answer choice may immediately look right. Be careful! Take a second to make sure that the other choices are not equally obvious. Don't make a hasty mistake. There are only two times that you should stop before checking other answers. First is when you are positive that the answer choice you have selected is correct. Second is when time is almost out and you have to make a quick guess!

Check Your Work

Since you will probably not know every term listed and the answer to every question, it is important that you get credit for the ones that you do know. Don't miss any questions through careless mistakes. If at all possible, try to take a second to look back over your answer selection and make sure you've selected the correct answer choice and haven't made a costly careless mistake (such as marking an answer choice that you didn't mean to mark). The time it takes for this quick double check should more than pay for itself in caught mistakes.

Beware of Directly Quoted Answers

Sometimes an answer choice will repeat word for word a portion of the question or reference section. However, beware of such exact duplication. It may be a trap! More than likely, the correct choice will paraphrase or summarize a point, rather than being exactly the same wording.

Slang

Scientific sounding answers are better than slang ones. An answer choice that begins "To compare the outcomes…" is much more likely to be correct than one that begins "Because some people insisted…"

Extreme Statements

Avoid wild answers that throw out highly controversial ideas that are proclaimed as established fact. An answer choice that states the "process should used in certain situations, if…" is much more likely to be correct than one that states the "process should be discontinued completely." The first is a calm rational statement and doesn't even make a definitive, uncompromising stance, using a hedge word "if" to provide wiggle room, whereas the second choice is a radical idea and far more extreme.

Answer Choice Families

When you have two or more answer choices that are direct opposites or parallels, one of them is usually the correct answer. For instance, if one answer choice states "x increases" and another answer choice states "x decreases" or "y increases," then those two or three answer choices are very similar in construction and fall into the same family of answer choices. A family of answer choices consists of two or three answer choices, very similar in construction, but often with directly opposite meanings. Usually the correct answer choice will be in that family of answer choices. The "odd man out" or answer choice that doesn't seem to fit the parallel construction of the other answer choices is more likely to be incorrect.

Special Report: How to Overcome Test Anxiety

The very nature of tests caters to some level of anxiety, nervousness, or tension, just as we feel for any important event that occurs in our lives. A little bit of anxiety or nervousness can be a good thing. It helps us with motivation, and makes achievement just that much sweeter. However, too much anxiety can be a problem, especially if it hinders our ability to function and perform.

"Test anxiety," is the term that refers to the emotional reactions that some test-takers experience when faced with a test or exam. Having a fear of testing and exams is based upon a rational fear, since the test-taker's performance can shape the course of an academic career. Nevertheless, experiencing excessive fear of examinations will only interfere with the test-taker's ability to perform and chance to be successful.

There are a large variety of causes that can contribute to the development and sensation of test anxiety. These include, but are not limited to, lack of preparation and worrying about issues surrounding the test.

Lack of Preparation

Lack of preparation can be identified by the following behaviors or situations:

Not scheduling enough time to study, and therefore cramming the night before the test or exam
Managing time poorly, to create the sensation that there is not enough time to do everything
Failing to organize the text information in advance, so that the study material consists of the entire text and not simply the pertinent information
Poor overall studying habits

Worrying, on the other hand, can be related to both the test taker, or many other factors around him/her that will be affected by the results of the test. These include worrying about:

Previous performances on similar exams, or exams in general
How friends and other students are achieving
The negative consequences that will result from a poor grade or failure

There are three primary elements to test anxiety. Physical components, which involve the same typical bodily reactions as those to acute anxiety (to be discussed below). Emotional factors have to do with fear or panic. Mental or cognitive issues concerning attention spans and memory abilities.

Physical Signals

There are many different symptoms of test anxiety, and these are not limited to mental and emotional strain. Frequently there are a range of physical signals that will let a test taker know that he/she is suffering from test anxiety. These bodily changes can include the following:

Perspiring
Sweaty palms
Wet, trembling hands
Nausea
Dry mouth
A knot in the stomach
Headache
Faintness
Muscle tension
Aching shoulders, back and neck
Rapid heart beat
Feeling too hot/cold

To recognize the sensation of test anxiety, a test-taker should monitor him/herself for the following sensations:

The physical distress symptoms as listed above
Emotional sensitivity, expressing emotional feelings such as the need to cry or laugh too much, or a sensation of anger or helplessness
A decreased ability to think, causing the test-taker to blank out or have racing thoughts that are hard to organize or control.

Though most students will feel some level of anxiety when faced with a test or exam, the majority can cope with that anxiety and maintain it at a manageable level. However, those who cannot are faced with a very real and very serious condition, which can and should be controlled for the immeasurable benefit of this sufferer.

Naturally, these sensations lead to negative results for the testing experience. The most common effects of test anxiety have to do with nervousness and mental blocking.

Nervousness

Nervousness can appear in several different levels:

The test-taker's difficulty, or even inability to read and understand the questions on the test
The difficulty or inability to organize thoughts to a coherent form
The difficulty or inability to recall key words and concepts relating to the testing questions (especially essays)
The receipt of poor grades on a test, though the test material was well known by the test taker

Conversely, a person may also experience mental blocking, which involves:

Blanking out on test questions
Only remembering the correct answers to the questions when the test has already finished.

Fortunately for test anxiety sufferers, beating these feelings, to a large degree, has to do with proper preparation. When a test taker has a feeling of preparedness, then anxiety will be dramatically lessened.

The first step to resolving anxiety issues is to distinguish which of the two types of anxiety are being suffered. If the anxiety is a direct result of a lack of preparation, this should be considered a normal reaction, and the anxiety level (as opposed to the test results) shouldn't be anything to worry about. However, if, when adequately prepared, the test-taker still panics, blanks out, or seems to overreact, this is not a fully rational reaction. While this can be considered normal too, there are many ways to combat and overcome these effects.

Remember that anxiety cannot be entirely eliminated, however, there are ways to minimize it, to make the anxiety easier to manage. Preparation is one of the best ways to minimize test anxiety. Therefore the following techniques are wise in order to best fight off any anxiety that may want to build.

To begin with, try to avoid cramming before a test, whenever it is possible. By trying to memorize an entire term's worth of information in one day, you'll be shocking your system, and not giving yourself a very good chance to absorb the information. This is an easy path to anxiety, so for those who suffer from test anxiety, cramming should not even be considered an option.

Instead of cramming, work throughout the semester to combine all of the material which is presented throughout the semester, and work on it gradually as the course goes by, making sure to master the main concepts first, leaving minor details for a week or so before the test.

To study for the upcoming exam, be sure to pose questions that may be on the examination, to gauge the ability to answer them by integrating the ideas from your texts, notes and lectures, as well as any supplementary readings.

If it is truly impossible to cover all of the information that was covered in that particular term, concentrate on the most important portions, that can be covered very well. Learn these concepts as best as possible, so that when the test comes, a goal can be made to use these concepts as presentations of your knowledge.

In addition to study habits, changes in attitude are critical to beating a struggle with test anxiety. In fact, an improvement of the perspective over the entire test-taking experience can actually help a test taker to enjoy studying and therefore improve the overall experience. Be certain not to overemphasize the significance of the grade - know that the result of the test is neither a reflection of self worth, nor is it a measure of intelligence; one grade will not predict a person's future success.

To improve an overall testing outlook, the following steps should be tried:

Keeping in mind that the most reasonable expectation for taking a test is to expect to try to demonstrate as much of what you know as you possibly can.
Reminding ourselves that a test is only one test; this is not the only one, and there will be others.
The thought of thinking of oneself in an irrational, all-or-nothing term should be avoided at all costs.
A reward should be designated for after the test, so there's something to look forward to. Whether it be going to a movie, going out to eat, or simply visiting friends, schedule it in advance, and do it no matter what result is expected on the exam.

Test-takers should also keep in mind that the basics are some of the most important things, even beyond anti-anxiety techniques and studying. Never neglect the basic social, emotional and biological needs, in order to try to absorb information. In order to best achieve, these three factors must be held as just as important as the studying itself.

Study Steps

Remember the following important steps for studying:

Maintain healthy nutrition and exercise habits. Continue both your recreational activities and social pass times. These both contribute to your physical and emotional well being.
Be certain to get a good amount of sleep, especially the night before the test, because when you're overtired you are not able to perform to the best of your best ability.
Keep the studying pace to a moderate level by taking breaks when they are needed, and varying the work whenever possible, to keep the mind fresh instead of getting bored.
When enough studying has been done that all the material that can be learned has been learned, and the test taker is prepared for the test, stop studying and do something relaxing such as listening to music, watching a movie, or taking a warm bubble bath.

There are also many other techniques to minimize the uneasiness or apprehension that is experienced along with test anxiety before, during, or even after the examination. In fact, there are a great deal of things that can be done to stop anxiety from interfering with lifestyle and performance. Again, remember that anxiety will not be eliminated entirely, and it shouldn't be. Otherwise that "up" feeling for exams would not exist, and most of us depend on that sensation to perform better than usual. However, this anxiety has to be at a level that is manageable.

Of course, as we have just discussed, being prepared for the exam is half the battle right away. Attending all classes, finding out what knowledge will be expected on the exam, and knowing the exam schedules are easy steps to lowering anxiety. Keeping up with work will remove the need to cram, and efficient study habits will eliminate wasted time. Studying should be done in an ideal location for concentration, so that it is simple to become interested in the material and give it complete attention. A method such as SQ3R (Survey, Question, Read, Recite, Review) is a wonderful key to follow to make sure that the study habits are as effective as possible, especially in the case of learning from a textbook. Flashcards are great techniques for memorization. Learning to take good notes will mean that notes will be full of useful information, so that less sifting will need to be done to seek out what is pertinent for studying. Reviewing notes after class and then again on occasion will keep the information fresh in the mind. From notes that have been taken summary sheets and outlines can be made for simpler reviewing.

A study group can also be a very motivational and helpful place to study, as there will be a sharing of ideas, all of the minds can work together, to make sure that everyone understands, and the studying will be made more interesting because it will be a social occasion.

Basically, though, as long as the test-taker remains organized and self confident, with efficient study habits, less time will need to be spent studying, and higher grades will be achieved.

To become self confident, there are many useful steps. The first of these is "self talk." It has been shown through extensive research, that self-talk for students who suffer from test anxiety, should be well monitored, in order to make sure that it contributes to self confidence as opposed to sinking the student. Frequently the self talk of test-anxious students is negative or self-defeating, thinking that everyone else is smarter and faster, that they always mess up, and that if they don't do well, they'll fail the entire course. It is important to decreasing anxiety that awareness is made of self talk. Try writing any negative self thoughts and then disputing them with a positive statement instead. Begin self-encouragement as though it was a friend speaking. Repeat positive statements to help reprogram the mind to believing in successes instead of failures.

Helpful Techniques

Other extremely helpful techniques include:

Self-visualization of doing well and reaching goals
While aiming for an "A" level of understanding, don't try to "overprotect" by setting your expectations lower. This will only convince the mind to stop studying in order to meet the lower expectations.
Don't make comparisons with the results or habits of other students. These are individual factors, and different things work for different people, causing different results.
Strive to become an expert in learning what works well, and what can be done in order to improve. Consider collecting this data in a journal.
Create rewards for after studying instead of doing things before studying that will only turn into avoidance behaviors.
Make a practice of relaxing - by using methods such as progressive relaxation, self-hypnosis, guided imagery, etc - in order to make relaxation an automatic sensation.
Work on creating a state of relaxed concentration so that concentrating will take on the focus of the mind, so that none will be wasted on worrying.
Take good care of the physical self by eating well and getting enough sleep.
Plan in time for exercise and stick to this plan.

Beyond these techniques, there are other methods to be used before, during and after the test that will help the test-taker perform well in addition to overcoming anxiety.

Before the exam comes the academic preparation. This involves establishing a study schedule and beginning at least one week before the actual date of the test. By doing this, the anxiety of not having enough time to study for the test will be automatically eliminated. Moreover, this will make the studying a much more effective experience, ensuring that the learning will be an easier process. This relieves much undue pressure on the test-taker.

Summary sheets, note cards, and flash cards with the main concepts and examples of these main concepts should be prepared in advance of the actual studying time. A topic should never be eliminated from this process. By omitting a topic because it isn't expected to be on the test is only setting up the test-taker for anxiety should it actually appear on the exam. Utilize the course syllabus for laying out the topics that should be studied. Carefully go over the notes that were made in class, paying special attention to any of the issues that the professor took special care to emphasize while lecturing in class. In the textbooks, use the chapter review, or if possible, the chapter tests, to begin your review.

It may even be possible to ask the instructor what information will be covered on the exam, or what the format of the exam will be (for example, multiple choice, essay, free form, true-false). Additionally, see if it is possible to find out how many questions will be on the test. If a review sheet or sample test has been offered by the professor, make good use of it, above anything else, for the preparation for the test. Another great resource for getting to know the examination is reviewing tests from previous semesters. Use these tests to review, and aim to achieve a 100% score on each of the possible topics. With a few exceptions, the goal that you set for yourself is the highest one that you will reach.

Take all of the questions that were assigned as homework, and rework them to any other possible course material. The more problems reworked, the more skill and confidence will form as a result. When forming the solution to a problem, write out each of the steps. Don't simply do head work. By doing as many steps on paper as possible, much clarification and therefore confidence will be formed. Do this with as many homework problems as possible, before checking the answers. By checking the answer after each problem, a reinforcement will exist, that will not be on the exam. Study situations should be as exam-like as possible, to prime the test-taker's system for the experience. By waiting to check the answers at the end, a psychological advantage will be formed, to decrease the stress factor.

Another fantastic reason for not cramming is the avoidance of confusion in concepts, especially when it comes to mathematics. 8-10 hours of study will become one hundred percent more effective if it is spread out over a week or at least several days, instead of doing it all in one sitting. Recognize that the human brain requires time in order to assimilate new material, so frequent breaks and a span of study time over several days will be much more beneficial.

Additionally, don't study right up until the point of the exam. Studying should stop a minimum of one hour before the exam begins. This allows the brain to rest and put things in their proper order. This will also provide the time to become as relaxed as possible when going into the examination room. The test-taker will also have time to eat well and eat sensibly. Know that the brain needs food as much as the rest of the body. With enough food and enough sleep, as well as a relaxed attitude, the body and the mind are primed for success.

Avoid any anxious classmates who are talking about the exam. These students only spread anxiety, and are not worth sharing the anxious sentimentalities.

Before the test also involves creating a positive attitude, so mental preparation should also be a point of concentration. There are many keys to creating a positive attitude. Should fears become rushing in, make a visualization of taking the exam, doing well, and seeing an A written on the paper. Write out a list of affirmations that will bring a feeling of confidence, such as "I am doing well in my English class," "I studied well and know my material," "I enjoy this class." Even if the affirmations aren't believed at first, it sends a positive message to the subconscious which will result in an alteration of the overall belief system, which is the system that creates reality.

If a sensation of panic begins, work with the fear and imagine the very worst! Work through the entire scenario of not passing the test, failing the entire course, and dropping out of school, followed by not getting a job, and pushing a shopping cart through the dark alley where you'll live. This will place things into perspective! Then, practice deep breathing and create a visualization of the opposite situation - achieving an "A" on the exam, passing the entire course, receiving the degree at a graduation ceremony.

On the day of the test, there are many things to be done to ensure the best results, as well as the most calm outlook. The following stages are suggested in order to maximize test-taking potential:

Begin the examination day with a moderate breakfast, and avoid any coffee or beverages with caffeine if the test taker is prone to jitters. Even people who are used to managing caffeine can feel jittery or light-headed when it is taken on a test day.
Attempt to do something that is relaxing before the examination begins. As last minute cramming clouds the mastering of overall concepts, it is better to use this time to create a calming outlook.
Be certain to arrive at the test location well in advance, in order to provide time to select a location that is away from doors, windows and other distractions, as well as giving enough time to relax before the test begins.
Keep away from anxiety generating classmates who will upset the sensation of stability and relaxation that is being attempted before the exam.
Should the waiting period before the exam begins cause anxiety, create a self-distraction by reading a light magazine or something else that is relaxing and simple.

During the exam itself, read the entire exam from beginning to end, and find out how much time should be allotted to each individual problem. Once writing the exam, should more time be taken for a problem, it should be abandoned, in order to begin another problem. If there is time at the end, the unfinished problem can always be returned to and completed.

Read the instructions very carefully - twice - so that unpleasant surprises won't follow during or after the exam has ended.

When writing the exam, pretend that the situation is actually simply the completion of homework within a library, or at home. This will assist in forming a relaxed atmosphere, and will allow the brain extra focus for the complex thinking function.

Begin the exam with all of the questions with which the most confidence is felt. This will build the confidence level regarding the entire exam and will begin a quality momentum. This will also create encouragement for trying the problems where uncertainty resides.

Going with the "gut instinct" is always the way to go when solving a problem. Second guessing should be avoided at all costs. Have confidence in the ability to do well.

For essay questions, create an outline in advance that will keep the mind organized and make certain that all of the points are remembered. For multiple choice, read every answer, even if the correct one has been spotted - a better one may exist.

Continue at a pace that is reasonable and not rushed, in order to be able to work carefully. Provide enough time to go over the answers at the end, to check for small errors that can be corrected.

Should a feeling of panic begin, breathe deeply, and think of the feeling of the body releasing sand through its pores. Visualize a calm, peaceful place, and include all of the sights, sounds and sensations of this image. Continue the deep breathing, and take a few minutes to continue this with closed eyes. When all is well again, return to the test.

If a "blanking" occurs for a certain question, skip it and move on to the next question. There will be time to return to the other question later. Get everything done that can be done, first, to guarantee all the grades that can be compiled, and to build all of the confidence possible. Then return to the weaker questions to build the marks from there.

Remember, one's own reality can be created, so as long as the belief is there, success will follow. And remember: anxiety can happen later, right now, there's an exam to be written!

After the examination is complete, whether there is a feeling for a good grade or a bad grade, don't dwell on the exam, and be certain to follow through on the reward that was promised...and enjoy it! Don't dwell on any mistakes that have been made, as there is nothing that can be done at this point anyway.

Additionally, don't begin to study for the next test right away. Do something relaxing for a while, and let the mind relax and prepare itself to begin absorbing information again.

From the results of the exam - both the grade and the entire experience, be certain to learn from what has gone on. Perfect studying habits and work some more on confidence in order to make the next examination experience even better than the last one.

Learn to avoid places where openings occurred for laziness, procrastination and day dreaming.

Use the time between this exam and the next one to better learn to relax, even learning to relax on cue, so that any anxiety can be controlled during the next exam. Learn how to relax the body. Slouch in your chair if that helps. Tighten and then relax all of the different muscle groups, one group at a time, beginning with the feet and then working all the way up to the neck and face. This will ultimately relax the muscles more than they were to begin with. Learn how to breathe deeply and comfortably, and focus on this breathing going in and out as a relaxing thought. With every exhale, repeat the word "relax."

As common as test anxiety is, it is very possible to overcome it. Make yourself one of the test-takers who overcome this frustrating hindrance.

Additional Bonus Material

Due to our efforts to try to keep this book to a manageable length, we've created a link that will give you access to all of your additional bonus material.

Please visit http://www.mometrix.com/bonus948/cdm to access the information.